FRAMES AND LENSES

FRAMES AND LENSES

Jenean Carlton, ABOC, NCLC
President, Carlton & Associates, LLC
Atlanta, Ga

The Basic Bookshelf for Eyecare Professionals

Series Editors: Janice K. Ledford, COMT • Ken Daniels, OD • Robert Campbell, MD

SLACK INCORPORATED 6900 Grove Road, Thorofare, NJ 08086

Publisher: John H. Bond
Editorial Director: Amy E. Drummond
Assistant Editor: Lauren Biddle Plummer

Printed in the United States of America

ISBN 1-55642-364-0

Published by: SLACK Incorporated
6900 Grove Road
Thorofare, NJ 08086-9447 USA
Telephone: 856-848-1000
Fax: 856-853-5991
World Wide Web: http://www.slackinc.com

Contact SLACK Incorporated for more information about other books in this field or about the availability of our books from distributors outside the United States.

Last digit is print number: 10 9 8 7 6 5 4 3 2 1

Dedication

This book is dedicated to my family,
with love and admiration.

Contents

Acknowledgments

Several people were instrumental in the writing of this book and deserve recognition. I would first like to thank my husband, Andrew, for his consistent support of my career and for his wealth of knowledge that includes superior writing skills and computer expertise. I would also like to thank my good friend and artist, Karen Redner, for her artwork. The technical graphics she created for this book are some of the best I have seen in print. Finally, I would like to express my sincere gratitude to my editor, Jan Ledford, whose writing ability, humor, and expertise in the ophthalmic field has been of tremendous support to me during this endeavor.

About the Author

Jenean Carlton, ABOC, NCLC, has 15 years experience in the optical field. She is a Georgia licensed optician. In addition to working as a dispensing optician, she has served as business manager for large public and private optical firms. She has been a featured lecturer at the Southeastern Conference of Optometry since 1991. Her articles on managing optical firms and opticianry have appeared in various periodicals, including the *Southern Journal of Optometry, EyeWear,* and *Primary Care Optometry News.* She currently runs a consulting practice in Atlanta, Georgia, specializing in optical business strategy, staff training, and development.

Introduction

The overall goal of this book is to provide a strong foundation of broad-based optical information for optometric and ophthalmic personnel new to the field of optics, frames, and lenses, while also functioning as a review for industry veterans.

Early in my career, I was fortunate to work with a highly skilled team of opticians who were eager to share their knowledge with me. Their selfless teaching assisted me in gaining a basic level of clinical knowledge to build upon. During those apprentice-level years it become apparent to me that I was part of a successful group of opticians who were constantly striving to master their skills while at the same time providing only the highest level of care for their patients.

Whether I am consulting or managing businesses, that level of enthusiasm for the industry has stayed with me, and I am grateful to those professional opticians who "set the standards of care" that remain so important.

Optical professionals should place paramount importance on their responsibility to patients. Patients trust us to guide them in making eyewear decisions that will meet or exceed their visual needs. This challenge requires that we maintain current knowledge of lens and frame materials, design, and manufacture. Such knowledge, combined with attention to aesthetics and the customer's lifestyle, allows the professional to create an excellent end product for the wearer.

In writing this book, I strive to share my optical knowledge and experience with readers in hopes that doing so will assist them in providing excellent care to their patients.

Jenean Carlton, ABOC, NCLC

The Study Icons

The Basic Bookshelf for Eyecare Professionals is quality educational material designed for professionals in all branches of eyecare. Because so many of you want to expand your careers, we have made a special effort to include information needed for certification exams. When these study icons appear in the margin of a series book, it is your cue that the material next to the icon (which may be a paragraph or an entire section) is listed as a criteria item for a certification examination. Please use this key to identify the appropriate icon:

OptA	optometric assistant
OptT	optometric technician*
OphA	ophthalmic assistant
OphT	ophthalmic technician
OphMT	ophthalmic medical technologist
LV	low vision subspecialty
Srg	ophthalmic surgical assisting subspecialty
CL	contact lens registry
Optn	opticianry*
RA	retinal angiographer

**Because these icons apply to the entire text, they will not appear anywhere within this text.*

Chapter 1

Frames

OptA

KEY POINTS

- Today's frames are a product of artists, craftspeople, and computer-aided design (CAD).
- Cellulose acetate (or zyl) is the most commonly used material for plastic frames.
- Monel is a corrosion-resistant alloy, and is the most prevalent material used for metal frames.
- Spectacle frames are made up of a frame front and two temples. The front contains two eyewires, a bridge, and endpieces (where the temples attach to the frame front).
- The basic rule of thumb for frame fitting is to select a frame that is opposite to the patient's facial shape.

Once a practitioner has completed the examination and prescribed corrective lenses, it is then necessary to assist patients in selecting ophthalmic frames that will:

- Securely hold the prescription lenses in place directly in front of the eyes
- Enhance the facial structure and appearance of the wearer
- Result in cosmetically appealing finished lenses

Highly skilled optical professionals realize that these frame-fitting requirements fall into their realm of responsibility. To successfully fit patients with prescription eyewear, each area must be addressed.

This section includes information pertaining to the manufacturing process of ophthalmic frames as well as common frame materials, frame styles, frame measurements, and styling techniques. Please refer to Chapter 4 for frame adjustment and fitting guidelines.

How Ophthalmic Frames are Manufactured

Factories throughout the world combine expert craftspeople and master artisans with computer-aided design (CAD) to create frames that will meet the cosmetic as well as functional demands of today's eyewear consumer.

Frame styles begin as sketches on paper and are perfected with CAD. Next, a prototype of the design is fabricated by hand to analyze the new style. If the frame is selected as a suitable model, master tools are created to manufacture parts of the frame via automation. Automated machinery allows the producer to make frame components quickly and uniformly. However, for any given frame there are between 60 to 90 steps in the manufacturing process, many of which are still done by hand.[1]

Metal Frame Manufacturing

Metal frame parts are manufactured from many different materials that are appropriate for certain parts of a frame. (Specific materials will be discussed later in this chapter.) For example, nose pad arms and endpieces are frequently made of nickel because it is a strong, yet pliable material. Because of this, nickel is a good material for parts that are frequently bent and adjusted.

Temples and Trim Pieces

There are several ways for a manufacturer to produce metal temples for a frame. One method is to stamp the temples out of a sheet of metal. Another is to begin with a metal cylinder and then stretch the metal to the desired length. After the metal cylinder is stretched, it is then molded into its final form. Some manufacturers have realized that the latter method results in temples that retain their shape longer than those that are simply stamped into shape. In addition, temples that begin as cylinders and are stretched first do not break easily when adjusted.

Trim pieces are decorative parts of a frame that are affixed to the upper eyewire or endpieces. Not only do they add decoration to a frame but they also add stability to the frame front. Trim pieces are frequently molded into shape and, like all frame parts, can be made even more ornate by using a multitude of coloration and/or decorative processes. Multiple drills are used in manufacturing facilities to install trim pieces to a frame.

Eyewires

Metal eyewires are made from either pure materials, such as titanium, or from metal alloys, such as stainless steel or Monel (Inco Limited, Toronto, Ontario). Eyewires are bent into shape using an eyewire curling machine. Small presses are used to add decorative treatments to metal frames, and hand crafted tooling or etching is often done to further enhance the appearance of the finished frame front.

Finishing

Many parts of a frame require soldering or spot welding to affix the parts securely into place, such as nose pad guard arms and bridges. In today's factories, spot welding done by hand has been replaced with sophisticated ultrasonic and laser soldering for improved adherence of the parts and for lasting durability.[1]

In the final production stages, metal parts are plated and galvanized by dipping them into a series of baths. This treatment ensures a durable and lasting finish on the frames. These coatings not only add luster and beauty but also extend the life of the frame.

The final coating applied to a frame is a protective finish. This is a clear coating that insulates the frame from external environmental factors such as perspiration and industrial atmospheres. Frame manufacturers use a series of tests to assure that frames withstand such threatening environments. These tests are:

- The Cass test that simulates a salt water and sea air environment
- The Kesternick test that duplicates an industrial atmosphere
- The Swiss University test that imitates the human body's acidic perspiration[1]

Parts are assembled by hand and serigraphy (silk screening) machines are employed to imprint the necessary frame information onto the parts. Relevant information, such as the frame model name or number, the sizes (front, bridge, and temples), and the color (which could be a number assigned to represent the color or a color name), is included on the frame. Once imprinted, the frames are packaged and prepared for shipping.

Plastic Frame Manufacturing

Cellulose acetate (or zyl) is the most commonly used material to manufacture plastic frames. It is stable, lightweight in nature, and offers virtually unlimited coloration possibilities. Zyl is created from a mixture of cottonseed fibers, wood flakes, plasticizers, and stabilizers. (Plasticizers and stabilizers keep the colors true and the material pliable.[2]) After the composite is produced, it is either compressed by heated rollers to form sheets of block zyl or made into a granular form that is melted and used to fabricate injection-molded frames.

Frame parts that are cut from slabs of block zyl have a tendency to be more durable than those made through injection-molded processes. However, milling parts from zyl slabs results in a high percentage of material waste and is more costly than producing frames through injection-molded procedures. In addition, sheets of zyl, unlike any other plastic material, may be laminated to further increase the uniqueness of the finalized look.

Frame Fronts and Temples

Frame fronts are milled out of small zyl slabs using pantographing machines. (Virgin zyl performs best. Virgin zyl means that the cellulose acetate used for the parts did not originate from scraps or left over zyl pieces.[1]) The pantographing machines first mill eyewires internally, then externally. Like metal frames, trim pieces are often added to further enhance the beauty and strength of a plastic frame.

Sometimes metal cores are added to plastic temples to provide strength and pliability. This feature is common with high quality plastic frames and makes for easier, longer-lasting adjustments.

Finishing

Decorative treatments are added in the final phase of ophthalmic frame production.

The individual talent and creativity of the artist determine the magnificence of a decorated frame. Professionally trained artists embellish metal frames with decorative treatments, such as baked-on transfer foil prints, hand-applied enamel, varnishes, inlaid stones, and tooled or etched eyewires. Because of the variety of treatments that are utilized to adorn metal frames, these are generally more ornate than plastic frames.

As with metal frames, the parts are assembled and stamped with all pertinent information regarding the model, size, and color, and are then packaged for shipping.

Tumbling

New frame parts (metal or plastic frames) are tumbled in wooden or metal crates with a variety of materials, such as pumice stone, walnut chips, and vegetable oils. This procedure smooths the rough edges of the frame parts while adding luster to the new styles. The tumbling process can take as long as 48 hours to complete. The radiance resulting from the tumbling process cannot be scratched or peeled off, particularly on plastic frames. High quality manufacturing processes, such as tumbling, become apparent by the feel of the frame. Frames that are tumbled for a long period of time feel smooth to the touch and are of a high luster.

OphA

Frame Materials

This section provides information about common frame materials used in the industry today. Probably the most difficult aspect of working with a frame is determining the material that the frame is made of. This is especially true for some of the new-age plastic materials. To properly handle the frame without damaging it during the adjustment process or when mounting lenses, it is immensely helpful to know this information. Manufacturers usually do not include the frame material (other than titanium, and even then we do not know the percentage of titanium in the model) as part of the information that is stamped onto the frame.

One way to handle this predicament is to realize that often venders group products together based on the material. Examples of such situations are Christian Dior by Safilo (Padua, Italy), many of these styles are made of Optyl (Safilo, Padua, Italy); SuperThin (Marchon, Melville, NY) makes stainless steel designs; Ti22 (Marcolin, Longarane, Italy) uses titanium; etc. Ask your venders for more detailed information about the materials used in their frame lines.

While it appears to be more common these days, it is still rare that a patient is allergic to a particular frame material. Most frame allergies occur as a response to frames made of nickel. An allergic reaction to nickel manifests as a burning sensation of the skin (where the frame touches) or as a rash. In many people, this can lead to an infection of the problem area if not treated.

At the point of sale, it is advantageous to ask if the patient has any known metal allergies. Adults who are allergic to nickel most often know this; however, children usually do not. (Costume jewelry is frequently made of nickel, and adults who are nickel-sensitive know if they have had problems with nickel-based earrings that caused their ears to itch or bleed. Sometimes even belt buckles made of nickel will cause a problem for the allergic wearer.)

Patients experiencing allergic reactions to their frames should choose a new style. (Hopefully the problem is detected early enough so the individual will not be charged for the new frame.) Suitable materials for individuals with nickel sensitivities are plastic frames, stainless steel (even though stainless steel is an alloy that includes nickel), and titanium. The material of choice is titanium (100% or close). However, some titanium frames offer a mere fraction of the pure metal and could incorporate nickel into the manufacturing process.

As a zyl frame ages (zyl itself will be discussed in detail later), the plasticizers that keep the frame pliable are secreted from the plastic material. This is especially true if the frame has been exposed to temperatures over 160 degrees (Fahrenheit), which could occur if the frame is left inside a car on a very warm day or if heated with a bead pan or air blower that exceeds this temperature. This is also why plastic frames become brittle and ashy in the nasal area and on the eyewires over time. The rare patient who has an allergic reaction to a plastic frame is most often having a reaction to the plasticizers that are emerging from the material due to age or excessive heat.[3] This is difficult to explain to a patient, especially one who has been wearing his or her plastic frame successfully for a long period of time without any problems.

Patients who have experienced this problem with plastic frames would do best to select a plastic frame made of propionate, polyamide, or Optyl. Propionate is a very strong plastic material ordinarily used for ultra-thin plastic styles due to its strength. Color is applied to propionate frames in the final processes as a series of overcoatings. Because it is coated on the surface of the material rather than within the material itself, it tends to "lock" in the plasticizers. Frames made of polyamide material do not incorporate any plasticizers in the manufacturing process. Optyl is a lightweight, hypoallergenic plastic material that has a "memory." When heated to 176 degrees, Optyl will return to its original shape. It is very strong and is not made with plasticizers, thus it does not pose allergy problems for a wearer.

Plastic Frame Materials

Cellulose Acetate (Zyl)

Cellulose acetate (or zyl) is a mixture of cottonseed fibers, wood flakes, stabilizers, and plasticizers. It is the most common frame material used today for manufacturing plastic frames.

Zyl is easy to adjust and has the unique ability to slightly reduce in size to accommodate a lens that is edged a bit small or to stretch to house a lens that is edged too large. As mentioned earlier, zyl lends itself well to coloration processes and the possibilities are essentially limitless. Frames are made of this material by one of two methods: either by milling or cutting the frames from block zyl sheets (slabs) or by injection-molded methods that make use of a granular form of the material.

Frames can be made from a single zyl slab or from slabs that are laminated together to result in a more unique product. Manufacturing frames from the pantographing method results in high quality, stable styles, but the process can be costly and wasteful due to the excess zyl that is forfeited during the procedure. (Pantographing machines are machines that mill or cut product from zyl slabs.)

If used in the granular form, zyl is first melted and then injected into frame molds. Frames produced from this type of technology are called injection-molded plastic frames. The process for manufacturing injection-molded plastic frames is less costly than the block zyl variety, and produces less waste. However, injection-molded frames tend to be less stable than those made from block zyl. Because of this, it is common to see injection-molded frames, as well as all zyl frames, coupled with metal temple cores for added strength.

Adjustment Tips

Before adjusting a zyl frame, heat the material (preferably only the area that is to be adjusted) either in a bead pan or with an air blower. The material is easy to work with and is not excessively heat sensitive. However, overheating the frame can cause irreversible damage. As with all frames, if using a bead pan, keep the frame in constant motion once it is immersed into the glass beads. Otherwise, burning or marring of the frame surface may result. If high-index lenses or other "soft" lens materials are mounted into the frame, try using a tissue between the frame and the beads to minimize the possibility of damaging the frame or the lenses. Bead-damaged lenses appear "dotted." This effect is called "orange peel" in the industry and can sometimes be reversed by dipping the lenses into the heated neutralizer for a few seconds. (*Note:* Using the neutralizer is not an option for anti-reflective coated lenses.) The best way to avoid damaged lenses is to remove the lenses from the frame before heating, use an air blower to heat the frame, or use a tissue between the glasses and the beads (as stated above).

Zyl frames are sensitive to some solvents, particularly acetone. When it is necessary to use acetone on a frame or lenses (as when removing progressive markings), first try using denatured alcohol. Also, use a cotton swab with the solution to minimize damaging the glasses. Be cautious when using acetone on all plastic frames, as it will damage and dull the material.

As zyl ages, the material becomes less flexible and can take on a whitish appearance, particularly in the bridge area and the eyewires. This can occur with time due to the loss of plasticizers (conditioners). When making lenses for an older zyl frame, it is always necessary to check the eyewires for cracks due to brittleness. Small cracks in the eyewires will most likely continue to crack when the lenses are inserted due to heating the frame and stretching the material. Inspecting old frames thoroughly before mounting new lens could save you the cost of a replacement frame, as well as lens and labor costs.

Mounting slightly oversized lenses into a zyl frame is easily accomplished by thoroughly heating the frame until it becomes very pliable and then carefully inserting the lenses into the eyewires. Use caution when heating a frame to this degree, as the heat may cause the hinges to become loose, and the eyewires sometimes have a tendency to "roll" when mounting oversized lenses. ("Rolled" eyewires generally appear on older zyl frames due to the loss of pliability in the material.) Also, larger sized lenses could cause the eyewires to split due to the stress on the material. The best solution for such a problem is to slightly edge the lenses down on a hand stone if qualified personnel and equipment are available.

Cellulose Propionate

Cellulose propionate is another plastic material used to produce injection-molded frames. Because it is lightweight and very strong it lends itself well to the production of ultra-thin and oversized frame styles. As mentioned earlier, the coloration process for propionate is done in the final processes and is applied over the material rather than as part of the substance. This tends to seal in the plasticizers, which makes it a good choice for patients who have had allergic reactions to plastic frames in the past and it also renders the frame more scratch resistant.

Propionate is very heat-sensitive and is damaged by temperatures over 105 degrees. Frames made of this material are best heated with an air blower to control the temperature. When using a bead pan, use low heat and remember to keep the frame in motion to avoid damaging the frame surface. Propionate does not stretch or shrink much, so it is important to size the lenses as one would for a "cold snap" frame. (The cold snap method of lens insertion is used for heat-sensitive frame materials and indicates that lenses are mounted without heating the frame. Lenses should be "edged to size" for mounting in plastic frames that are heat sensitive.)

Using alcohol and/or acetone on propionate will most likely cause permanent damage. For the best results, remove the lenses before attempting to clean off any lens markings with solvents.

Carbon Fiber Graphite

Carbon fiber graphite manufactured by Marchon (Melville, NY) is a lightweight material (about one fourth the weight of zyl and metal) that consists of a carbon compound (no less than 30% carbon by weight) and a textile fiber called ceramic whisker. Once united, these materials make for a lightweight and stable product with a very high tensile strength. Frames made with this material are produced through injection-molded methods. Due to its strength, it is useful for applications other than eyewear, such as golf clubs, tennis racquets, skis, and automobile bumpers.[2]

Carbon fiber graphite is a very dark and fibrous material. In fact, if you break one of these frames into pieces (it is hard to do because the material is so strong), it looks dark gray and thread-like. Because of its darkness, transparent colors are not available and baked-on colored enamels are applied over the material. Carbon fiber graphite frames are available in a wide variety of solid colors or with mottled color patterns.

This material is minimally affected by heat, so it is of little help to heat the frame before adjusting. Most carbon fiber graphite frames have eyewires with screws, so the lenses are edged as they are for a metal frame which makes lens insertion easy. Carbon fiber graphite frames are not particularly sensitive to solvents such as alcohol or acetone.

Polycarbonate

Polycarbonate is used in the manufacturing of bulletproof glass and crash helmets. In the eyecare industry, polycarbonate is used for ophthalmic lenses and sport and safety frames. It is the most impact-resistant material available for frame or lens production. When safety is an issue, polycarbonate is always the material of choice. Individuals who play sports or who have potentially dangerous occupations or hobbies should be educated about the safety advantages of polycarbonate frames and lenses.

Frames made of polycarbonate are manufactured through injection-molded technology and are limited to safety and sport styles. Sport frames made from this material are usually clear and have soft nose and temple pads that attach to the frame for added comfort.

Polycarbonate is inherently soft, which is why it absorbs impact without shattering. However, even though the material is virtually shatterproof, it is very easy to scratch. While most polycarbonate lenses are manufactured with a tough, scratch-resistant coating to protect the lens surface, this protective coating is not available for polycarbonate frames. To minimize scratching, patients should be instructed in proper handling and cleaning techniques for these frames. Cleaning frames made from polycarbonate is similar to cleaning polycarbonate lenses; rinse the material well with water and use a mild cleaning solution such as dish washing detergent, if needed. Polycarbonate frames or lenses are easily scratched if wiped when dry.

Polycarbonate is rigid, making it difficult to adjust frames made of this material. For the best results, the frame should fit well on the initial fitting. Adjustments are limited and heating the material will not add much flexibility. Lenses should be edged for a "cold mount," as the frame will not stretch when heated. Like other plastic materials, polycarbonate is also solvent sensitive; acetone and alcohol should not be used on this material.

Polyamide

Another transparent material that lends itself to injection-molded frame technology is polyamide. Polyamide is a type of nylon that is very strong and lightweight in nature, this makes it a perfect material for fabricating frames that are very thin and durable. Polyamide is easily tinted and is available in a wide range of colors. Plasticizers are not used in the production of polyamide frames so it is a good choice for individuals who are sensitive to some types of plastics.

Care should be taken when adjusting frames made of polyamide. This material is very heat sensitive and frequently reduces in size when heated (shrinkage results when using temperatures over 230 degrees on these frames.)[3] Always edge lenses to size when working with polyamide and cold snap the lenses into the frame. While the heat sensitivity of this frame material is a drawback, it can actually be beneficial if the lenses are edged slightly too small. In this case, heat the frame with the lenses inserted and the frame will reduce in size to meet the dimensions of the lenses.

Optyl

Optyl is a plastic frame material that is hypoallergenic, lightweight, and keeps its finish over time. Frame manufacturers commonly use this substance to create stylish, durable frames that are available in a multitude of colors and with elaborate decorate treatments. Plasticizers are not used in the manufacturing process of this resin so it is a good choice for patients who are sensitive to some types of plastic frames.

Optyl is a lasting, durable material known for returning to its original shape when thoroughly heated. This can be of great value if the frame is in need of an adjustment. (The material is not easily damaged by excessive heat in the bead pan or by an air blower.) To return the frame to its original shape, simply heat the frame and set it aside to cool. Do not insert the frame into water, the frame will return to its original shape while cooling. While this feature is often an advantage to the dispenser, it could cause problems if the goal is to alter the frame shape. For example, if you have slightly stretched the bridge of an Optyl frame to better fit a patient, the frame will return to the original shape when heated to a high temperature.

For best results, only heat the portion of an Optyl frame that is to be adjusted. This can be accomplished by making "mounds" of glass beads in your bead pan and inserting only the part of the frame that needs adjusting into these stacks. An air blower is also effectively used to heat Optyl frames if the air is directed to the specific part(s) of the frame that needs adjusting. Optyl is a brittle material. To avoid breakage, always heat the frame thoroughly, even when performing the simplest of alterations.

Nylon

Nylon is a virtually unbreakable, hypoallergenic frame material that, in today's market, is mostly used for injection-molded sunglasses as well as men's frame styles. It does not respond much to heat, which makes it nearly impossible to alter the adjustment. (When heating nylon, use a tissue to hold the frames as the material holds heat and will burn your fingers.) Nylon frames are usually very dark in color.

Nylon neither shrinks nor stretches, so it is very important to edge the lenses for the exact size. It is also beneficial to occasionally soak these frames in water overnight, as the material has a tendency to dry out (which results in an ashy appearance).

Metal Frame Materials

Metal spectacle frames are manufactured from either pure metals such as titanium, or from metal alloys such as Monel. The following information will familiarize you with materials that are used in manufacturing today's metal frames.

Monel

Monel is a combination of nickel and copper. This material is the most common substance used to produce metal designs. Monel is a strong, stable material that also lends itself to making nose pad arms, bridges, and endpieces. It is resistant to corrosion and is economical for use in the frame manufacturing process.

Nickel

Nickel (Ni on the periodic table) is an element that is strong and generally bends without breaking, which makes it suitable for endpieces and nose pad arms. Nickel is also utilized with other metals to form alloys that are used in the fabrication of spectacle frames, such as stainless steel.

Patients are sometimes allergic to nickel products. Nickel allergies present as a skin rash anywhere that the frame touches the face or as a burning sensation on the skin. When working with a patient with a known nickel allergy, suggest a frame material that is hypoallergenic.

Nickel Silver

Also known as alpaca or German silver, nickel silver is an alloy made of copper, zinc, silver, and nickel. It is a strong, rigid material that is suitable for hinges, endpieces, bridges, and decorative trims. This material is brittle, which makes it a poor choice for frame fronts or thin parts. However, when used as an inner core for plastic temples, it improves the durability of the product and allows for longer-lasting adjustments.[2]

Phosphorous Bronze

Also called phosphor-bronze, phosphorous bronze is an alloy comprised mostly of copper. Copper is a flexible material which makes it a good choice for frame styles requiring thin temples; however, adjustments can be a problem because of the "springy" characteristic of the material. This material is susceptible to tarnishing, yet has a lustrous shine when polished.[3]

Stainless Steel

Stainless steel frames are very popular because the material is strong even in thin, streamlined applications. This metal is an alloy comprised of manganese, nickel, iron, and chromium. Extreme temple adjustments can be a challenge because stainless steel is a rigid, springy material; anything more than simple adjustments can be problematic. Frames made of this metal should fit relatively well on the initial fitting.

Stainless steel is very resistant to corrosion and makes a good frame material for people who work outdoors or who have had problems with frame corrosion due to perspiration. Even though stainless steel has a small amount of nickel in the alloy, patients with known metal sensitivities are not likely to have problems with this material.

Titanium

Titanium (Ti) is a naturally occurring element that is highly corrosion-resistant and is incredibly lightweight (specific gravity is 4.54). The eyewear industry has realized the value of this material for comfort and durability, and a multitude of titanium frames (of varying percentages of the material) are available. To date, it is difficult to know the percentage of titanium that is in a given style. This, of course, is of great importance to the wearer as well as to the practitioner, particularly if the wearer is allergic to other metals and is purchasing a titanium frame to avoid allergic skin reactions. This issue is currently being addressed by the industry and will hopefully result in manufacturing guidelines for titanium products.

Because it is difficult to retrieve from the earth, and is such a rigid material to work with (special tools are often needed to manufacture or decorate this material), frames made of titanium can be costly.

Aluminum

Many years ago, aluminum frames were tremendously popular. You probably have seen those antique silver, cat eye-shaped aluminum frames with inlaid jewels and beautiful etchings.

Aluminum (Al) is a lightweight element abundant in the earth's crust (specific gravity is 2.69). This makes it even lighter than titanium (4.54). However, it is a rigid material that is difficult to adjust. Not many aluminum frames are made today due to the availability of more advanced materials.

Rarely someone may enter the office needing an adjustment on an aluminum frame. These frames use the type of nose pads that are clamped onto the nose pad guard arms. Carefully remove the old nose pad by inserting a screwdriver underneath the metal clamps to loosen the pad. When replacing the pads with new ones, be sure to clamp the new pads on tightly by using needle-nose pliers to flatten them into place.

Beryllium

Beryllium (Be) is an element used in conjunction with other metals, such as copper, to form alloys used in the frame manufacturing process. When mixed with copper it forms a springy material that is well suited for temple production. Beryllium alone is a strong material, but unfortunately it is costly.[2]

Cobalt

Cobalt (Co) is an element that is used as part of an alloy to make a very strong and non-corrosive frame material. Due to its higher cost, it is primarily used as a stabilizing interior metal on high quality frames. It offers a highly polished finish and is often used in thin frame designs.

OphA

Frame Styles

Whether plastic or metal, ophthalmic frames are available in many different styles. Types of frames available include full frame, combination frame, semi-rimless, full rimless or drill mount, and half-eyes (Figure 1-1).

A full frame has eyewires of either plastic or metal materials that completely surround the ophthalmic lenses.

A combination frame merges metal eyewires with plastic temples or vice versa. This union of materials is popular with many venders and in many different materials.

Semi-rimless, which is commonly referred to as a rimless frame or rimless mount, is very popular in the current frame market. The upper half of the eyewire is made from either a plastic or metal material while the lower portion consists of a nylon cord. Lenses for this type of frame are grooved to hold the cord in place. Because these lenses must be grooved, it is not recommended to use a semi-rimless frame style for farsighted (hyperopic) patients with a power of over +3.00 D per lens. Plus lenses are thicker in the center and wafer thin on the edge. To successfully groove lenses for a semi-rimless frame, the lens must have a considerable amount of edge thickness. High plus lenses are "built up" in the center to result in enough edge thickness to effectively groove the lenses. Because of this, plus lenses are generally thicker in a semi-rimless frame.

Full rimless or drill mount frame styles consist of only temples, endpieces, and a bridge piece. The lenses are suspended by screws that connect the lenses to the bridge and endpieces or by clips that holds these parts into place. The lenses in these frame styles are often beveled or faceted for added ornamentation. Again, plus lenses over +3.00 D are not recommended for this design

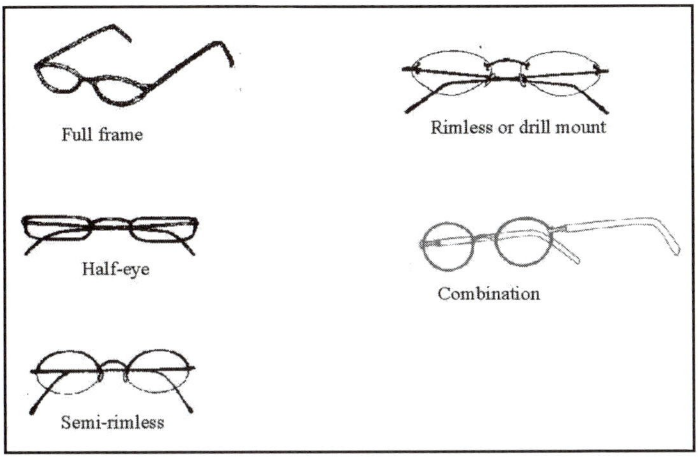

Figure 1-1. Frame styles.

because of the need to increase the degree of edge thickness. The edge thickness of lenses used for this design are sometimes slightly increased so that the lenses will not chip or crack easily while wearing or during an adjustment.

Half-eye frames are used for patients with a near-vision-only correction. These patients need corrective lenses to clearly see objects at a reading distance. (This distance is routinely 16 inches away from the patient, but the power can be altered by a practitioner for different focal ranges.) Half-eye frames can be made of either plastic or metal materials. They are also available in semi-rimless styles. Semi-rimless styles make particularly successful half-eye frames because the nylon cord is at the top of these frames rather than at the bottom. The frame is worn low on the nose so that the patient may look over them for easy distance viewing, then simply drop the gaze for near viewing through the lenses. Semi-rimless half-eye styles are easier to use because the wearer looks over an unobtrusive nylon cord rather than looking over a thicker eyewire material such as plastic.

Parts of a Frame

OphA

Spectacle frames, either metal or plastic, are made up of three main components: a frame front and two temples (Figure 1-2). The front is that portion of a frame that contains two eyewires, some type of a bridge, and endpieces. The bridge joins the eyewires, and the endpieces attach the temples to the frame front. Temples are needed to securely hold the front and prescription lenses in place.

Frame Front

The frame front has either a sculpted bridge (as in plastic frames) or a bridge device that is attached to the frame (such as nose pads). The bridge is an important part of the frame because it connects the two eyewires and it supports most of the weight of the spectacles on the patient's nose.

Types of Bridges

Bridges for Plastic Frames

Plastic frames incorporate a saddle, modified saddle, keyhole, or adjustable bridge (nose pads) (Figure 1-3).

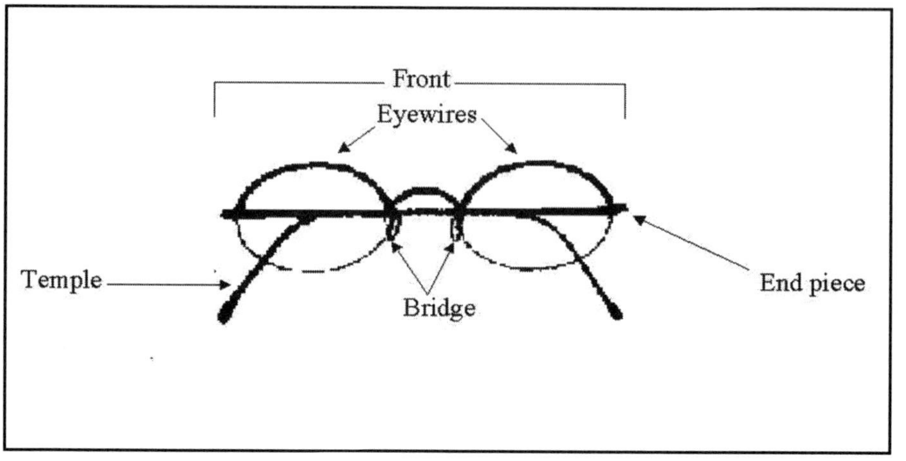

Figure 1-2. Parts of a frame.

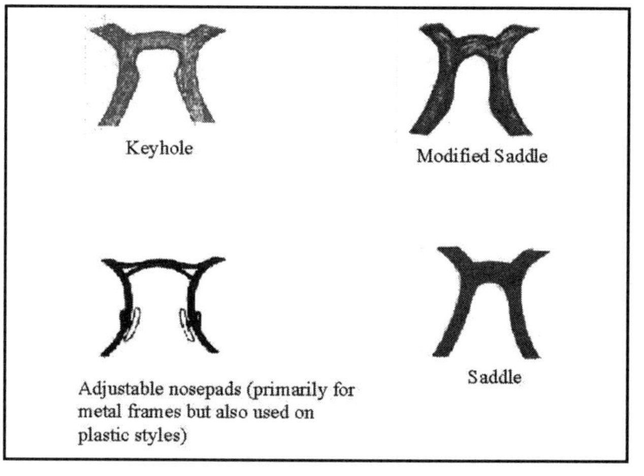

Figure 1-3. Bridge styles for plastic frames.

A saddle bridge is designed to evenly distribute the weight of the spectacles on the top as well as sides of the nose. This type of bridge is best suited for patients who have expressed sensitivity to frames with nose pads. A modified saddle is similar to the saddle design except it also offers built-up areas on either side of the bridge. This modification is helpful when fitting a patient with a very narrow nose, as the built up areas can often be heated and brought in slightly for a better fit. The keyhole bridge is another good selection for patients who have a very thin bridge, or who are sensitive to pressure on the top of the nose (such as someone who has had surgery or is prone to sinus problems).

Some plastic frames are available with adjustable nose pads. This is especially beneficial for patients who desire a zyl frame but because of their facial features (a very thin bridge or high cheekbones) are best suited for a metal frame. Frames with nose pads allow for a good fit; however, the weight of the glasses is balanced solely on the nose pads. This can sometimes cause discomfort for patients, particularly those needing heavy, high-powered lenses. When adjusting plastic frames with nose pads, avoid heating the area where the nose pad guard arm is inserted into the plastic material. Heating this area could cause the plastic material to expand, which may result in the arm dislodging from the frame front.

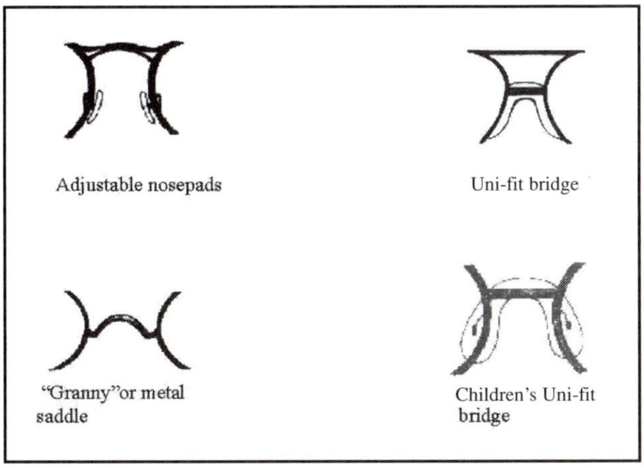

Figure 1-4. Bridge styles for metal frames.

Bridges for Metal Frames

Metal frames are constructed with adjustable nose pads, a uni-fit bridge, or a saddle bridge (Figure 1-4). As mentioned earlier, adjustable nose pads balance the entire weight of the glasses on two pads. Nose pads are available in acetate (these are often referred to as "hard" pads) or in very soft silicon. Silicon pads are far superior to acetate because they slightly "grip" the skin and tend to hold the glasses in the proper position better than the acetate variety. Rarely does anyone have a reaction to silicon material. (However, a silicon allergy presents as a rash or as red, inflamed skin. Persons who are sensitive to silicon should use acetate pads.) Silicon pads are available in several different sizes and shapes (10 mm round to regular 21 mm). They offer maximum comfort and should be replaced as needed.

A uni-fit bridge resembles and functions like a saddle bridge on a plastic frame. It is usually attached to the metal bridge by tiny screws and evenly distributes the weight of the glasses on the wearer's bridge. Uni-fit bridge styles are a good choice for safety frames (because safety lenses tend to be heavier due to the rules governing center thickness) and for high-powered prescription dress lenses. Unfortunately, frames with this bridge design are mostly limited to men's styles, safety eyewear, and children's frames. Children are good candidates for uni-fit bridge styles because their facial structure is not fully developed, and this design enables them to wear comfortable, well-fit eyewear.

Uni-fit bridges are most often made of silicon. Some even have a metal insert that allows for a long-lasting, stable adjustment. Some metal frames are made with an acetate uni-fit bridge. After time, this may prove to be a problem as the material may shrink slightly due to drying. This situation can result in a bridge that will not stay affixed to the frame. When this is the case, it is necessary to order a new bridge for the frame from the manufacturer.

The saddle bridge has made a recent comeback on trendy metal styles. It is a curved metal bridge that supports the weight of the glasses mostly on the top of the bridge. It is not recommended for patients requiring heavy, high-powered lenses as it may cause discomfort due to the weight of the glasses.

Temples

There are five basic temple designs used in frame manufacturing:

1. Skull temples
2. Library temples

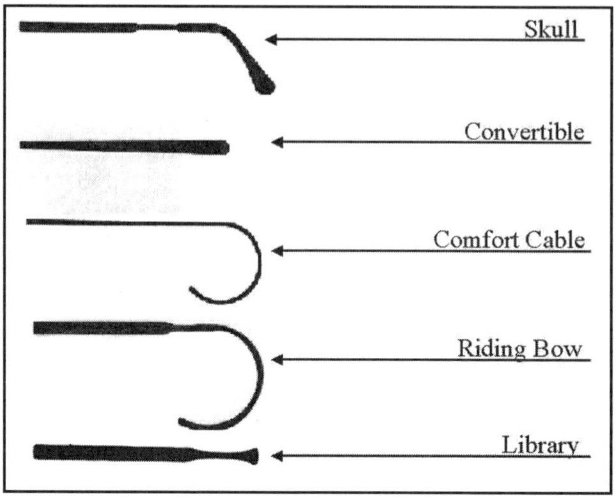

Figure 1-5. Temple styles.

3. Convertible temples
4. Comfort cable temples
5. Riding bow temples (Figure 1-5)

The most commonly used temple designs are the skull and comfort cable.

Skull temples are adjusted to closely follow the structure of the patient's ear. The best temple adjustments always begin with a heated temple end. The bend of the temple should be a smooth curve and never "hooked." Properly adjusted skull temples follow the curve of the wearer's ear and do not put excessive pressure on the ear lobe or mastoid process (located behind the ear). Pressure in these areas can result in pain and discomfort for the wearer.

Library temples are designed to fit straight back so that they hug the patient's skull. This temple style is commonly seen on half-eye reader frames and on military aviator frames. The straight-back design of the temples enables the wearer to quickly position the frame on and off the face. For optimum results, bow the temples in slightly so the tension will hold the frame in position against the wearer's head.

Convertible temples can be worn adjusted straight back (like library temples) or behind the ear (like skull temples). This temple design offers patients either choice for wearing comfort.

Comfort cable temples are routinely used for children's frames and safety and sport styles. Comfort cables are metal coil temples that are very springy. These temples are quite effective at holding a frame securely in place and are a good choice for some active occupations such as an electrician or a mechanic; they are also beneficial for people (such as children) who could possibly lose or damage their eyewear because of their activities. Comfort cables can be shaped to fit either very tightly or loosely, depending on the adjustment. To loosen the coil, simply bend the cable in its reverse direction; forming the coil into a smaller circle tightens the adjustment.

Cable temples are often encased in a flexible plastic temple cover for added comfort. If needed, this jacket can be replaced. Simply cut off the old cable jacket with chapel pliers and insert the cable into a new covering. Using an air blower, slightly heat the new sheath until it shrinks to the shape of the coil.

Riding bow temples are also used for children's, sport, and safety frames. This style is similar to the comfort cable temple because it is shaped to curl around the back of the ear. However, riding bow temples are constructed from plastic materials rather than metal coils. The rigid plastic material can make these temples a challenge to fit. Even in the most skilled of hands, they can be difficult to adjust into a smooth curve. For best results, heat these temples thoroughly before shaping.

Frame Measurements

The boxing system is the optical industry's preferred means of obtaining necessary frame and lens measurements. (Please see Chapter 3 for a full discussion of the boxing system.)

Even though manufacturers stamp the length of the temples directly onto the frame parts, sometimes this information is mistakenly taken off (with solvents) or is worn off. If this happens, the length of the temple can be determined by first heating the temple end and straightening the bend. After this is done, use a millimeter ruler to measure from the beginning of the temple (do not include the endpiece) to the end of the temple cover. The resulting measurement is the length of the temple in millimeters.

Frame Selection

The best frame for a patient complements his or her facial structure, requires minimal adjustments, and will securely hold the lenses in place. Also, because of its shape and size, the chosen frame will positively affect the cosmetic appearance of the prescription lenses.

Frame Styling

Frame styling begins by obtaining a mental image of the finished lens. (Please see more n this topic in Chapter 4.) This is a technique that comes with experience and is quite beneficial in selecting the appropriate frame for a given prescription. The size and the shape of the frame greatly affect the overall cosmetic appearance of the finished prescription lenses.

The best way to control the finished look is to first imagine the thickness and curves of the lenses. For instance, a high minus lens will be thick on the edges and thin in the center; compounding this prescription with a high cylinder correction will add extra thickness to an area of the lens corresponding to the cylinder axis. A good choice for such a prescription is a small, rounded frame. Selecting a frame that meets this criteria will result in lenses that are as thin as possible; selecting a large, angular frame would result in much thicker and heavier lenses for the same correction.

Determining the Facial Shape

Determining the patient's facial shape is the next step. There are essentially seven facial shapes:

1. Oval
2. Round
3. Triangle
4. Long
5. Square
6. Inverted triangle
7. Diamond (Figure 1-6)

Deciding the shape of someone's face can be a difficult task. It often takes serious observation, and sometimes a patient's face may take on a combination of several shapes. One trick to determine someone's facial shape (or your own) is to have the patient trace his or her face on a mirror with a piece of soap. (This is easily cleaned off and makes the facial shape decision easi-

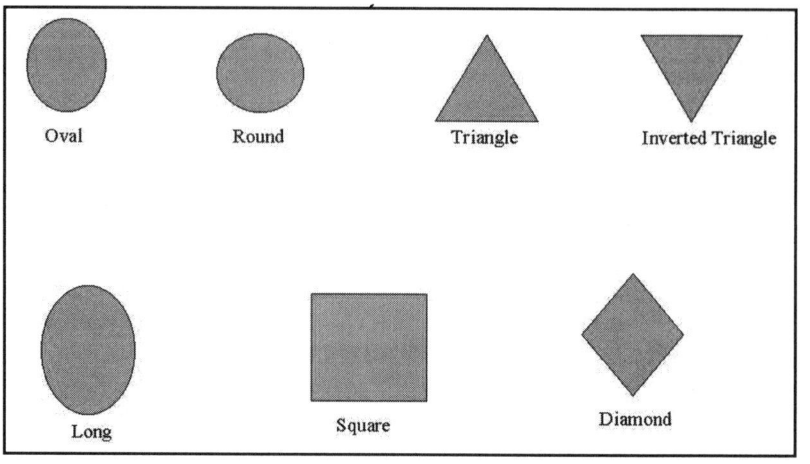

Figure 1-6. Common facial shapes.

What the Patient Needs to Know

- Your eyewear dispenser has been specially trained to help you select frames and lenses that will be functional and attractive.
- Factors to consider when choosing a frame include facial shape, facial features, and overall coloring.
- Not every prescription can be fit into every frame. The thickness of some lenses may mean that they will not fit into certain frames.
- If you have a special need or condition (such as sensitivity across the bridge of the nose or an allergy to a certain material), please tell your dispenser.
- If you work with or around electricity, it is best to select a plastic frame since metal conducts a current.

er for you and the patient.) The basic rule of thumb for frame fitting is to select a frame that is opposite to the patient's facial shape. This results in a balanced look for the wearer and accentuates his or her positive features. Choosing a frame that is the same shape as the face emphasizes the facial shape. For instance, a round shaped face is made to appear less round by selecting an angular frame; choosing an oval frame would accent the roundness of the face.

Using Frames to Balance Facial Proportions

Oval-shaped faces usually look good in any frame shape. This is the only facial shape that enjoys this advantage. Rounded faces look best in angular frames; frames that offer a high temple attachment are a plus. Square faces look best in round or oval shaped frames; the goal here is to avoid angles. Faces that are long in shape take on a more balanced look by selecting styles with a small "B" measurement. (The "B" measurement is the deepest vertical measurement of the eyewire. See The Boxing System in Chapter 3 for further information.) The smaller "B" measurement makes the face appear shorter. Triangle-, inverted triangle-, and diamond-shaped faces are all very angular and appear softer in frames with oval or rounded designs. Rimless frames, as well as frames with delicate colors and features, are also a good choice for this group as they soften the overall appearance of the wearer's face.

Selecting a Lens Material and Multifocal Design

At this point it is necessary to select a lens material and multifocal style (if required). Sometimes the lens material may dictate the frame style needed for a patient. An example would be glass lenses. Glass lenses are not suitable for mounting into rimless or drill mount frame styles. Likewise, progressive lenses are of little benefit if edged for a trendy frame with a very small "B" measurement. (Recently some lens manufacturers have addressed this problem by producing progressive lenses with a shorter corridor that are good choices for frames with smaller "B" measurements. Ask your lens representatives for more information about these lenses.) Selecting the lens material and the multifocal design early on in the frame selection process saves valuable time and ensures that the patient will achieve greater satisfaction with the finished eyewear.

Discuss Frame Materials

As mentioned earlier in this chapter, some patients may have allergies or sensitivities to some materials used in the metal or plastic frame production process. It is important to ask patients during the frame selection process if they have any known allergies to plastics or metals.

Blending the information obtained in each section narrows down the final frame selection. It is important to understand that most often there is not a frame that will meet each objective perfectly. The goal is to meet or exceed the patient's visual expectations while also enhancing the overall appearance of the patient and the lenses.

References

1. Marchon & Marcolin. *Frame Materials and Frame Manufacturing* (handout).

2. Weber JM, Humphrey FJ, Rutherford W. Lesson No. 2: *Modern Ophthalmic Frame Materials.* Melville, NY: Marchon & Marcolin; 1991.

3. Disanto M. *Ophthalmic Spectacle Frame Materials.* Bowie, Md: National Academy of Opticianry; 1991.

- Oval shaped face looks good in everything
- Rounded - angular frames.
- Square: round or oval shape. (avoid angles)
- Triangle, - inverted triangle & diamond shaped appear softer in oval or rounded frames (rimless, delicate color.

Chapter 2

Lenses

KEY POINTS

- A spectacle lens consists of a transparent material that has two polished, opposing surfaces with the ability to focus light rays in an expected manner.
- The base curve of a spherical lens is ground on the front curve of the lens. Likewise, the base curve of spherocylindrical lenses (lenses that correct astigmatism) ground in minus cylinder (where the cylinder is ground on the backside of the lens) is also on the front surface of the lens.
- The best and least distorted vision through an ophthalmic lens is obtained by matching the patient's visual axis with the optical center of the lens.
- Single vision lenses correct vision for one focal length. Bifocal lenses correct vision at two distances, usually with a prescription for distance vision at the top of the lens and a segment at the bottom of the lens for close work. A conventional trifocal lens has a distance portion, an intermediate segment (usually calculated for 30 inches away, generally half the bifocal power), and a bottom segment to correct vision at 16 inches away.
- Safety lenses must have a minimum lens thickness of 3.0 mm (except lenses of +3.00 D or more, which must have a minimum thickness of 2.5 mm). They must also have the initials of the laboratory that manufactured them etched into the upper portion of the lenses.
- CR-39 (Pittsburgh Plate Glass Industries, Pittsburgh, PA) is the most common lens material used today.
- High index lenses are made of denser materials than conventional lens materials, producing thinner and lighter lenses.

OphT

Optical Principles

Before discussing various types of lens materials and lens designs, it is important to understand the basics of how lenses work. An ophthalmic lens, whether plastic or glass, is manufactured from translucent materials. (Light traveling through a nontransparent medium would scatter light, making it difficult to see.) A spectacle lens consists of a transparent material that has two polished, opposing surfaces with the ability to focus light rays in an expected manner. (For a full discussion on optics, please see Basic Bookshelf title *Optics, Retinoscopy, and Refractometry.*)

CL

The Electromagnetic Spectrum

The electromagnetic spectrum is an orderly arrangement of all known radiant energy. It ranges from the incredibly small cosmic gamma rays that are measured in nanometers, to the ultra-long alternating current rays that are measured in miles or kilometers (Figure 2-1). All rays or wavelengths of the electromagnetic spectrum surround us each day. However, we are only capable of seeing those wavelengths between 400-760 nm (some references state that the visible spectrum begins at 380 nm). These wavelengths comprise the visible spectrum and are perceived by the human eye because they stimulate the photoreceptors of the retina.

Sir Isaac Newton determined that white light is comprised of many different colors of light by conducting a series of tests. Newton's tests consisted of repeatedly directing a thin beam of light at an angle through a prism. Each time he directed the beam of light through the prism, a band of colored lights was projected onto the test screen (Figure 2-2.) Time and time again, the order of the colored bands proved to be consistent. Newton called the resultant band of colored lights the "spectrum" and the break up of white light into these colored components "dispersion."[1]

CL

OptA

Refraction

The power of an ophthalmic lens is determined by the speed of light through the material and the difference between the lens's front and back curve. Light is refracted (or bent) by a medium (or material) when the speed at which the light is traveling is slowed or increased due to the density of the medium. For instance, light traveling through air is slowed when it strikes the surface of a high-index lens. When the ray emerges from the opposite side of the lens and is once again traveling through air, it will angle upward due to the change in speed, because light travels faster in air than through the lens (Figure 2-3).

CL

OptA

Index of Refraction

The index of refraction is a ratio obtained by dividing the speed light travels through a specific material into the speed light travels through air. Light travels through air at a rate of 186,000 miles per second.

$$\frac{\text{Speed of light in air}}{\text{Speed of light in material}} = \text{Refractive index}$$

Light travels slower through some materials than others, depending on the density of the material. The denser the material, the slower light travels through it. The slower that light travels through a specific material, the higher the material's refractive index and the greater its refracting ability (Table 2-1).

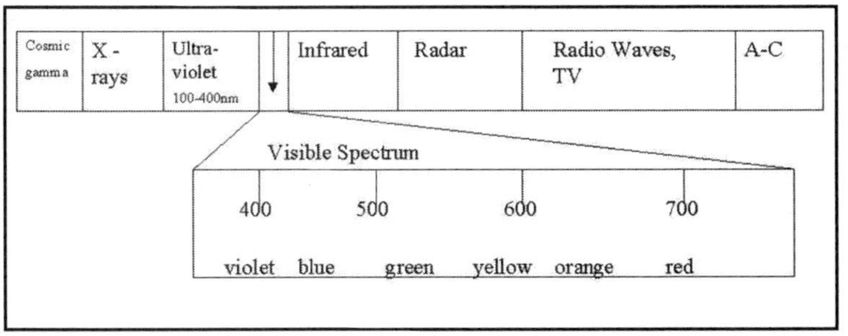

Figure 2-1. The visible spectrum consists of electromagnetic wavelengths that stimulate the retina and are between 400nm-760nm.

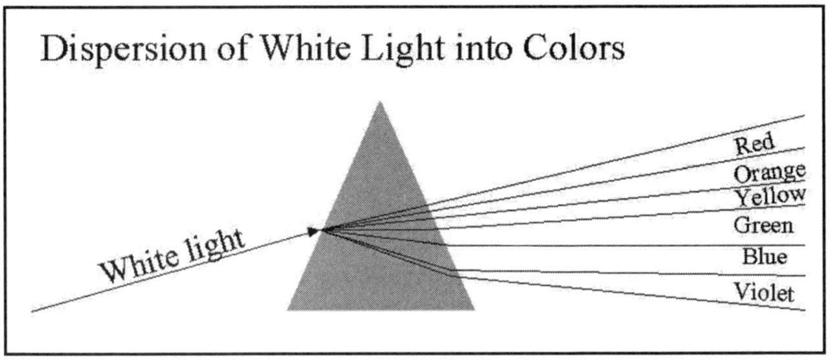

Figure 2-2. Chromatic aberration occurs when white light is broken into its spectral components.

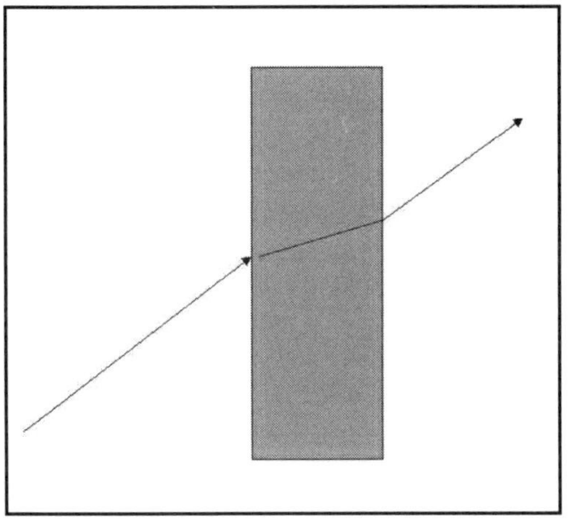

Figure 2-3. Light traveling through a lens.

Table 2-1
Index of Refraction for Common Lens Material

Material	Index
CR-39	1.498
Glass, crown	1.523
Spectralite (SOLA Optical USA, Petaluma, Calif)	1.537
High index 1.56 (resin)	1.556
Polycarbonate	1.586
High index 1.60 (resin)	1.60
High index 1.66 (resin)	1.66
Glass, barium crown	1.616

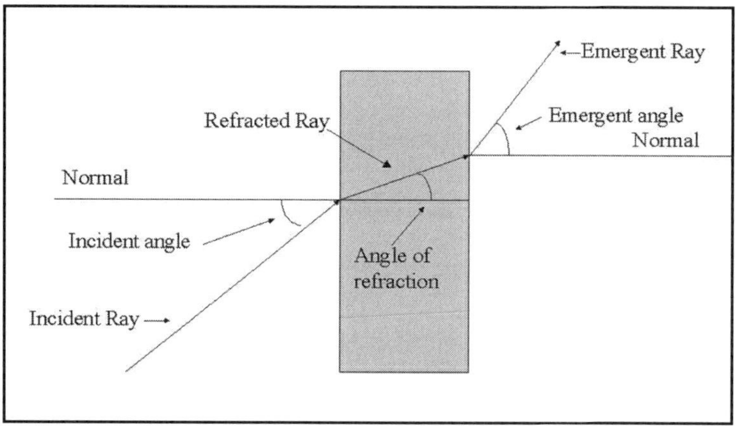

Figure 2-4. Snell's Law of Refraction.

High-index materials bend or refract light in the same manner as conventional materials, but with less mass due to the density of the material. High-index materials are denser than the conventional lens materials that cause light to travel at a slower rate. This slower rate of travel ultimately allows the lens to refract light in the same manner as the conventional material, but with less mass. Because of this, patients are able to appreciate thinner, lighter weight lenses that refract light in the same manner as conventional lens materials.

CL

Snell's Law of Refraction

In 1621, a Dutch astronomer and mathematician named Willebrord van Roijen Snell developed a theory of how light travels through a transparent substance. This theory is known today as "Snell's Law of Refraction." Although Snell did not publish his theory of refraction (it was later published by French mathematician and philosopher René Descartes as "Descartes' Law of Sines"), Snell's Law of Refraction is still used to explain how light is refracted by an ophthalmic lens (Figure 2-4).

Snell's Law explains that the constant relationship between the angle of incidence (the angle which is created between oblique light rays entering the medium and normal light rays), the angle of refraction (the angle created between the refracted light ray and normal light rays), and the index of refraction determine the ultimate refractive ability of the lens. Snell's Law of Refraction is the basis of all ophthalmic lens and ophthalmic instrument design.[1]

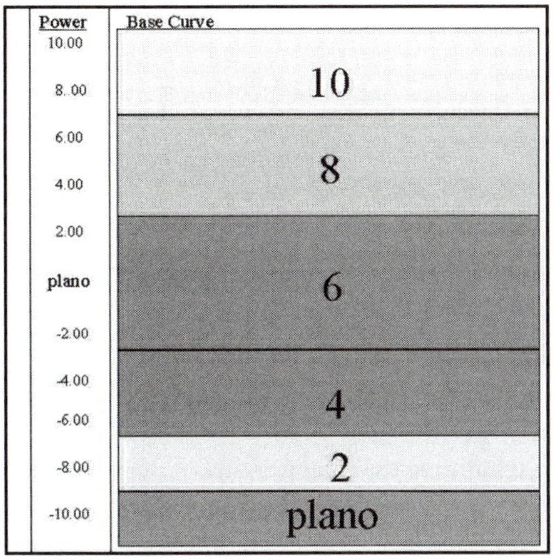

Figure 2-5. Example of a base curve chart.

Understanding Base Curves

OptA OphA

Every ophthalmic lens has a beginning or base curve. The base curve of a lens is easily determined by using a lens clock or lens measure (See Chapter 3). Base curves have a numeric value and are in either plus or minus form. For example, the base curve of a lens could be a low number (curves which are flat in nature), such as plano, 0.50, 2.00, 4.00, or 6.00. The base curve could also be a higher number, indicating a steeper curve, such as 8.00, 10.00, 12.00, or 14.00.

Base curves can be either even or odd numbers. Generally, lenses with odd base curves tend to be aspherically designed lenses. Lenses of even base curves are usually made of common materials and designs, such as CR-39 or regular glass. (These are all discussed later.)

All curves of an ophthalmic lens, as well as the resultant lens power, are dependent on the base or front curve. The base curve of a spherical lens is ground on the front curve of the lens. Likewise, the base curve of spherocylindrical lenses (lenses that correct astigmatism) ground in minus cylinder (where the cylinder is ground on the backside of the lens) is also on the front surface of the lens. The stronger curve on the backside of a spherocylindrical lens is called the cross curve, and the weaker curve is the toric base curve.

Manufacturers produce base curve selection charts to assist optical professionals in choosing the appropriate base curve for a given prescription (Figure 2-5). The suggested base curves will minimize unwanted peripheral problems and produce the best cosmetic appearance for the prescription, while also providing optimum vision. Base curves for a specific lens power may vary from vendor to vendor depending on each manufacturer's fabrication process.

Often times, a practitioner may state to "match the old base curve" on a prescription. It is important to use caution when opting for the old base curve, especially if the patient has experienced a significant change between the old and new prescription. However, if a patient wears a high-powered lens and has not experienced a change in the prescription, it is wise to specify the original base curve on the new order.

The total nominal power of a lens is determined by the difference between the front and back curves (Figure 2-6). For example, if we give the front surface of a lens the variable P1 (P= power), and the back surface P2, we can determine the total power of the lens, PT, by adding P1 and P2. Our formula is: P1 + P2 = PT where P1 = front curve, P2= back curve, and PT= total power.

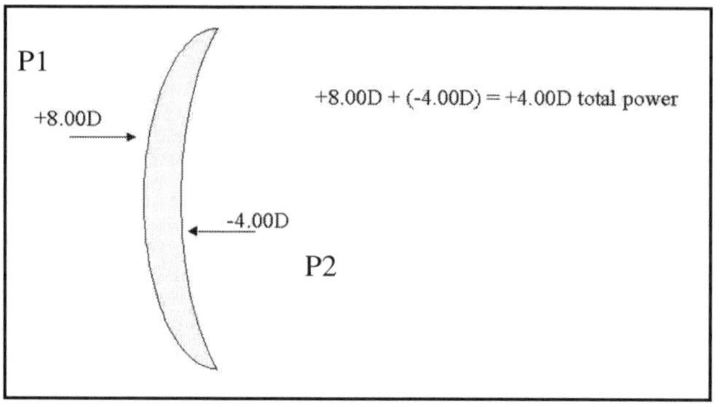

Figure 2-6. The nominal power of a lens is the difference between the front and back curves.

For example, let's imagine that we are trying to determine the total nominal power of a lens with a front curve of +10.00 and a back curve of -6.00. Our formula is +10.00 + (-6.00) = +4.00. The total power of the lens is +4.00 D. However, we could use several numeric combinations to obtain this same lens power of +4.00 D. We could have a front curve of +8.00 with a back curve of -4.00, where +8.00 + (-4.00) = +4.00. (These are, in fact, the usual curvatures for a +4.00 D lens ground on an 8 base.) The possible combinations are endless; however, manufacturers select the appropriate base curve to produce the best overall vision for the wearer.

Chromatic Aberration and Abbe Value

Lens materials, especially those with a high refractive index, often cause color dispersion or problems of chromatic aberration. Chromatic aberration occurs when white light is divided into its spectral color components. Patients often describe this as seeing color fringes or a bright yellow band on the edge of objects viewed through the periphery of the lenses.

Generally, selecting a high index material that offers a lower refractive index than the original material can eliminate or significantly minimize chromatic aberration. Selecting a close-fitting frame that results in minimal decentration also helps to alleviate this problem. However, the most accurate means of selecting the best lens material for the patient is to choose a high index medium that offers a high Abbe value.

The Abbe value (first described by Ernest K. Abbe, a German optical physicist) indicates the ability of a lens material to purely refract white light without chromatic aberration. It is sometimes referred to as the Nu value, and runs between 1 and 100. The closer the Abbe number is to 100, the more efficient the lens material. A high Abbe number indicates that the material is not likely to cause chromatic problems when viewing objects through portions of the lenses other then the optical center. A low Abbe number indicates that the material could cause chromatic distortion problems (Table 2-2).

OptA OphA LV CL

Visual Axis

The best and least distorted vision through an ophthalmic lens is obtained by matching the patient's visual axis with the optical center of the lens (Figure 2-7). (The visual axis is an imaginary line from a viewed object in the visual field to the fovea centralis of the retina. The fovea centralis is a small recession in the retina that produces our sharpest vision.) When alignment is accurate, the patient looks directly through the optical center of the lens without the presence of any unwanted vertical or horizontal prism.

Table 2-2
Abbe Values of Common Lens Materials

Material	Index
Glass, crown	59
CR-39	58
Spectralite	47
High index 1.56 (resin)	39
High index 1.60 (resin)	37
High index 1.66 (resin)	32
Polycarbonate	31
High index glass	25

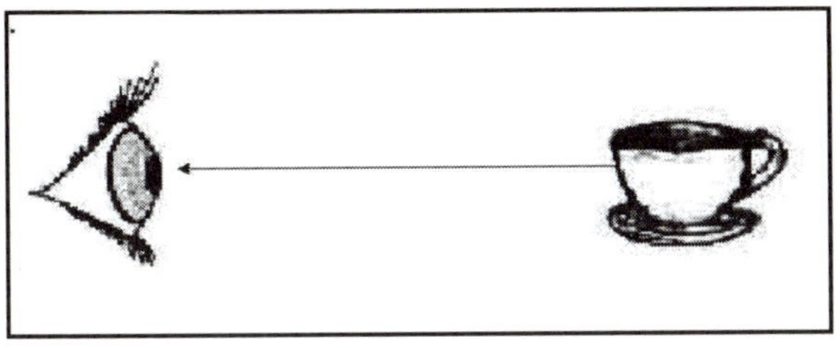

Figure 2-7. The visual axis is an imaginary line from a viewed object in the visual field to the fovea centralis of the retina.

With a lens of low power, a slight misalignment between the visual axis and optical center might not even be noticed by the patient. However, when considering lenses of moderate to significant power (+/-4.00D), images viewed through the periphery of the lens are not as clear as those viewed through the optical center. Images seen through the periphery could appear malformed due to chromatic aberration, unwanted cylinder aberration, or distortion.

Lens Types

Lenses are classified as spheres, cylinders, or prisms.

Spheres

Spheres are lenses that appear to have been sliced from the side of a round ball. A spherical lens has the same power throughout the lens. When viewed through a lensometer, the mires of a spherical lens look the same when rotating the axis wheel. (This is an easy way to confirm that the lens is spherical. The lensometer is covered in Chapter 3.) Spherical lenses are either convex (plus powered lenses), or concave (minus powered lenses) (Figure 2-8).

Plus powered lenses are convex lenses that magnify objects. They curve outward, more on the front of the lens than on the back. The thickest portion of the lens is in the center, and the edges are thin. Plus powered lenses converge light behind the lens to bring the image into focus on the retina. A plus lens can be considered as two prisms that are placed base-to-base (Figure 2-9). Patients requiring plus powered lenses have a refractive error called hyperopia and are commonly referred to as being "farsighted."

Minus lenses are concave lenses that minify objects. They are deeply curved on the back of the lens. The thickest portion of a minus lens is the edge and the thinnest area is the center. Minus lenses diverge light in front of the lens in order to focus the image on the retina. A minus lens can

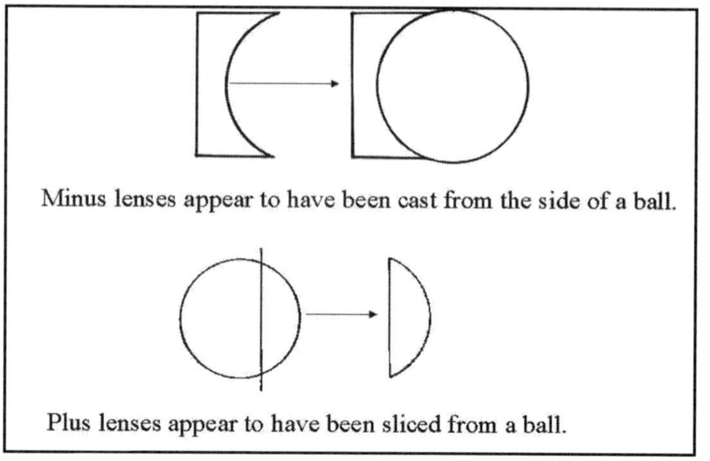

Figure 2-8. Spherical lenses.

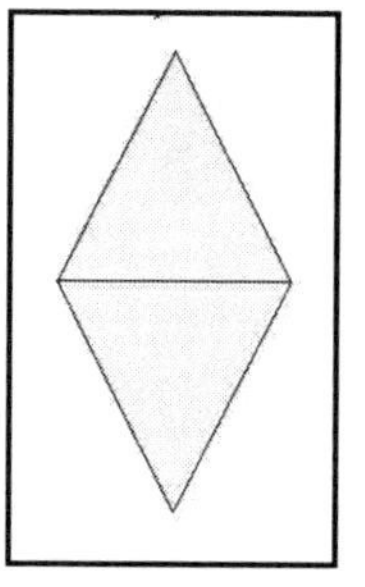

Figure 2-9. Plus lenses are two prisms placed base-to-base. (The thickest part of a prism is the base.)

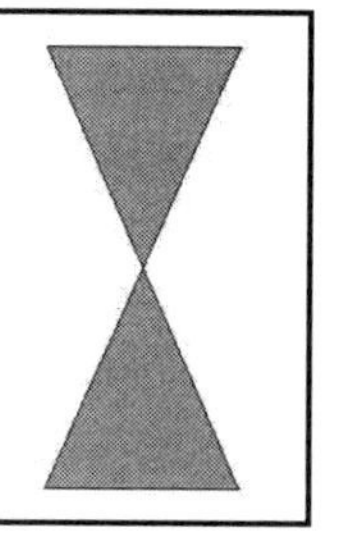

Figure 2-10. Minus lenses are two prisms placed apex-to-apex. (The thinnest part of a prism is the apex.)

be thought of as two prisms that are positioned apex-to-apex (Figure 2-10). Patients requiring a minus lens have a refractive error called myopia and are commonly referred to as being "nearsighted."

Cylinders

Lenses with cylinder correction appear to have been sliced from the side of a football (Figure 2-11). These lenses are not round; they appear to be obliquely shaped. The angle of the obliqueness depends on the meridian (direction) in which the cylinder correction lies. A cylinder focuses light in a thin line. If the lens is rotated, the focused line of light rotates as well.

When reading a cylindrical lens with the lensometer, one set of mires will appear sharp and clear when the lens is on axis. However, rotating the axis wheel will result in mires that are broken when the lens is off axis. This is an easy way to determine that the lens is, in fact, cylindrical.

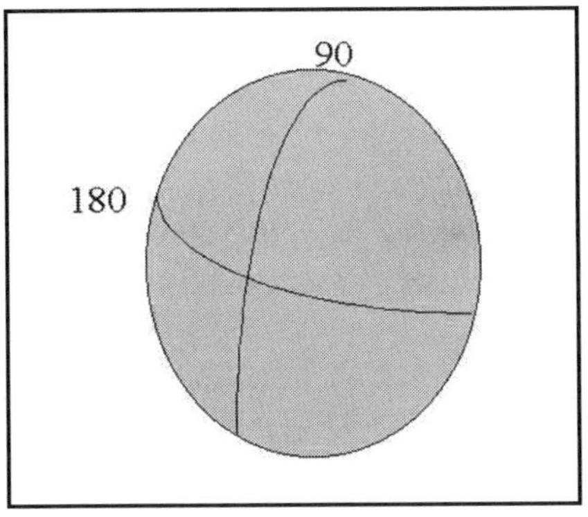

Figure 2-11. Cylindrical lens. The 90 degree mark denotes the vertical meridian and the 180 mark indicates the horizontal meridian.

Cylindrical lenses correct a refractive error called astigmatism. Patients with astigmatism have blurred vision caused by an irregularly curved cornea, crystalline lens, or other meridian of the eye. Left uncorrected, objects are blurred or nonspecific to patients with this problem. Practitioners correct astigmatism by prescribing cylindrical lenses that are curved in the opposite direction as the obliquely curved meridian that is causing the refractive error. By prescribing the cylinder correction in the opposite direction as the irregularly curved meridian of the eye, the astigmatism is neutralized and the patient appreciates clear vision.

Cylinder lenses can be plano-cylinder, which means the lenses have only a cylindrical component and no spherical power (example: plano – 1.00 x 090). They can also be spherocylindrical. Spherocylindrical lenses have a sphere correction as well as a cylinder correction (example: -1.00 – 2.25 x 075). All cylindrical lenses will have an axis which indicates the direction of the correcting curve.

Patients who have not had astigmatic correction in the past or who have experienced a change in their cylinder correction sometimes complain of noticing a "swimmy" sensation in the periphery of the new lenses. They may also state that objects appear to be malformed, such as a line appears bent or a tabletop seems slanted. Even the slightest change in cylinder correction can cause sensitive patients to react to the new power.

After wearing the lenses for a few days most patients become accustomed to the new correction and have good visual acuity. It is a good idea to re-inspect all lenses that are causing problems for a patient; this should be done immediately at the time of the complaint. Some offices have established a triage form to define the problem.

Prisms

Prisms are triangular in shape, thicker at the base and thinner at the apex. Light travels through the apex and is directed towards the base; images are displaced toward the apex (Figure 2-12). As mentioned earlier, spherical lenses can actually be thought of as a combination of prisms. (A minus lens is two prisms placed apex-to-apex, and a plus lens is two prisms placed base-to-base.) Prism correction is prescribed in prism diopters. One prism diopter displaces the image of an object one meter away by one centimeter.

Prisms are prescribed to correct eye muscle imbalances. Patients with eye muscle imbalances cannot appreciate a single fused image because the muscles of each eye do not work in harmony with one another (Figure 2-13). The image provided by each eye is so different that the two images cannot be fused.

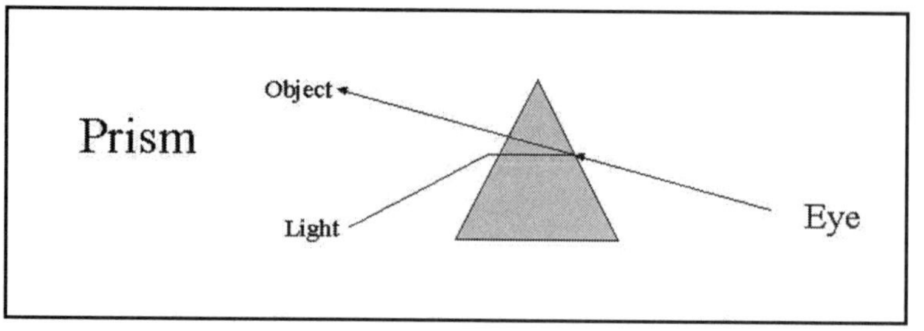

Figure 2-12. A prism bends light toward its base and objects appear displaced toward the apex. One prism diopter displaces an object 1 cm at a distance of 1 m from the eye.

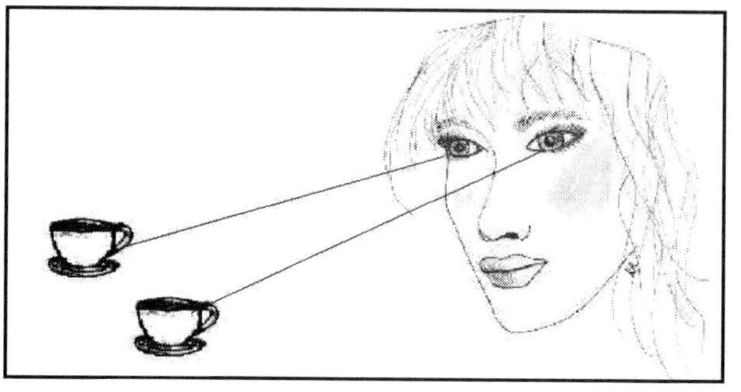

Figure 2-13. Patients with eye muscle problems cannot achieve one fused image.

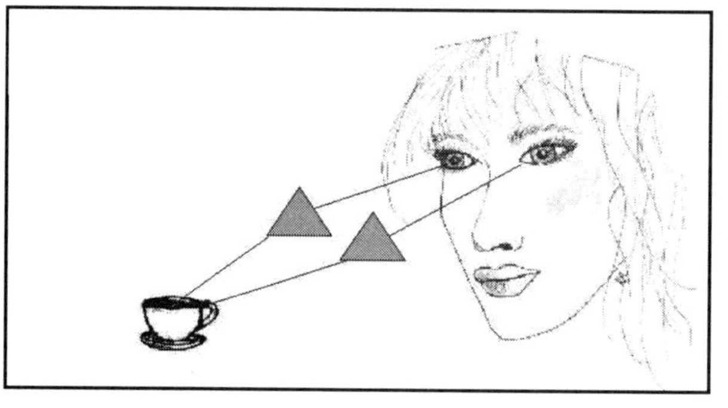

Figure 2-14. Prism correction allows the patient to appreciate one fused image (schematic).

Stereopsis is real, three-dimensional vision that is only obtained when both eyes work precisely together to create one fused image. Lenses with prism correction help the patient to achieve stereopsis by giving the patient a sensory alignment of the two images without affecting the motor alignment of the out-of-balance eye muscles. The object of regard is perceived as being displaced (Figure 2-14). This can be done by moving the optical center of the lens into a new position or by grinding the prism right into the lens. The degree of the displacement depends on the strength of the prism. (One 1.00 D of prism creates a slight displacement while 6.00 D of prism results in a significant displacement.) This is discussed in more detail in Chapter 3.

Prism correction displaces objects in a particular direction as defined by the position of the prism base. This position is determined by the physician according to the patient's muscle imbalance. Prisms can be prescribed as Base In (BI), Base Out (BO), Base Up (BU), or Base Down (BD). Base In and Out correct horizontal muscle imbalances; Base Up and Down correct vertical imbalances. An example of a prescription with prism correction is:

OD +2.00 sph. 4.00 D BU
OS +2.00 sph.

In the above prescription, all of the prism correction is ground into the right lens. This would result in the right lens being much thicker than the left. The difference in thickness would be apparent at the top of the right lens because the base of the prism is up. Altering the prescription so that the prism is divided between the two lenses would result in a more cosmetically appealing look, as well as balancing the weight of the lenses. The new prescription would look like this:

OD +2.00 sph. 2.00 D BU
OS +2.00 sph. 2.00 D BD

In this case, the right lens would be slightly thicker at the top and the left lens would be slightly thicker at the bottom. (*Note:* Before altering a prescription in any way it is necessary to first consult with the prescribing doctor.)

A prism can also be prescribed as compound prism. This type of prescription would correct for both horizontal and vertical imbalances. An example of a compound prism prescription is:

OD +2.00 sph. 2.00 D BU, 1.00 D BO
OS +2.00 sph. 2.00 D BD, 1.00 D BO

Single Vision, Bifocal, and Multifocal Lenses

OptA OphA

Single Vision Lenses

LV

Single vision lenses correct vision for one focal length. (Focal length is the distance at which the lens focuses an object that is 1 meter away from the lens.) They could be prescribed for distance vision only or for near vision only. They could even be calculated for intermediate vision (approximately 30 inches away from the eye), which would be particularly helpful for someone like a musician who sometimes needs assistance in seeing objects at an intermediate distance. However, due to accommodation, patients under 40 can often times wear their single vision lenses for multiple tasks.

Accommodation is the ability of the crystalline lens to change its shape in order to produce clear vision at closer viewing distances. For example, the crystalline lens becomes more rounded in shape (which creates a greater degree of plus power) when viewing objects at near. Likewise, it becomes flatter and thinner (which creates more minus power) to clearly view objects at a distance. When we are young, the eye has a wide range of focusing power. However, as we age this range slowly decreases, making it necessary for the majority of us to depend on near vision glasses for close work. The gradual loss of accommodation is called presbyopia. Patients with presbyopia require single vision reading glasses or bifocal lenses (discussed next) to assist them when viewing objects at a close range.

Bifocals

LV

Bifocal lenses correct vision at two distances, usually with a prescription for distance vision at the top of the lens and a segment at the bottom of the lens for close work. Most often the bifocal segment is calculated for viewing objects 16 inches away from the wearer's eye. Unless specified, the optical center is customarily ground 3 mm above the segment line.

Bifocal segments are available in many designs and sizes (Figure 2-15). There are round segments called Kryptok bifocals, as well as flat-top. When it comes to a lined segment, flat-top segments are more widely used today than rounded designs.

Round segments are available in 22 or 24-mm sizes, and flat-top bifocals are made in 25, 28, or 35-mm sizes. The size of the chosen segment depends on the occupation or hobbies of the indi-

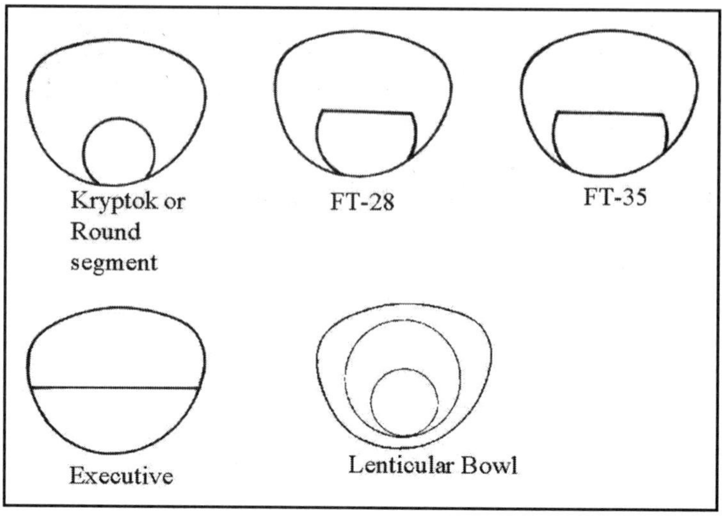

Figure 2-15. Bifocal styles.

vidual patient. Persons such as draftsmen or architects would require wider reading fields (due to the scanning nature of their close work) than patients who wear their glasses for occasional light reading.

The powers in the top and bifocal segments can be altered for different focal ranges. For instance, the top portion of the lens could correct for intermediate use, which would be helpful to someone who had difficulty seeing the computer screen clearly, while the bifocal segment still corrected for near vision. Or, the top portion of the lens could correct for distance and the bifocal segment could correct for intermediate vision. (*Note:* In this instance the bifocal would need to be raised higher than is standard practice to minimize discomfort for the wearer. Segment placement will be discussed later, in Chapter 3.)

To guarantee that the bifocal segment performs in the desired capacity, ask your patients to measure their working distance in inches and provide this information to the prescribing doctor. This will result in increased satisfaction for the patient, fewer lens remakes for the office, and less chair time for the physician.

LV

Trifocals

Trifocal lenses have three viewing distances or segments. A conventional trifocal lens has a distance portion, an intermediate segment (usually calculated for 30 inches away, generally half the bifocal power), and a bottom segment to correct vision at 16 inches away. Unless specified, the optical center for trifocal lenses is generally ground 3 mm above the trifocal segment line. There are many different trifocal lens designs in the marketplace (Figure 2-16).

Like bifocals, trifocal lenses can be prescribed to correct vision at varying distances. A pilot might need a trifocal lens that would correct vision for distance, the instrument panels, and near. Once again, by measuring the distance between the specific work area and the eye, the patient is able to report the accurate working distance to the practitioner.

Occupational Segments

Occupational lenses meet the visual demands of patients, such as electricians, who need to view close objects overhead clearly while also offering regular distance and near vision (Figure 2-

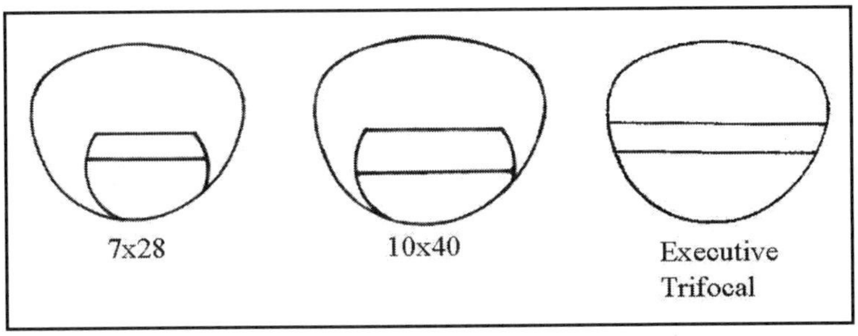

Figure 2-16. Trifocal styles.

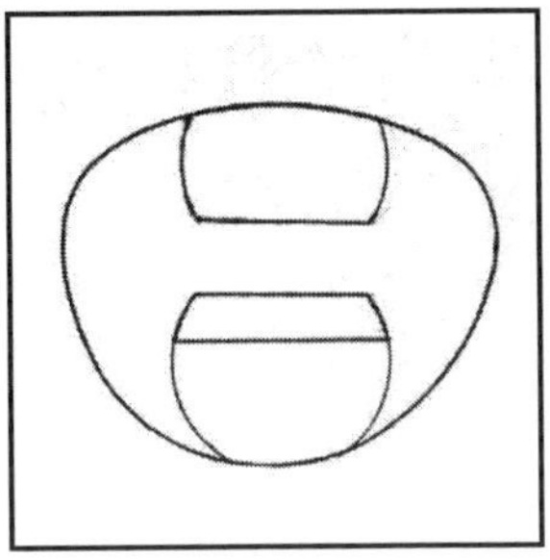

Figure 2-17. Occupational lens.

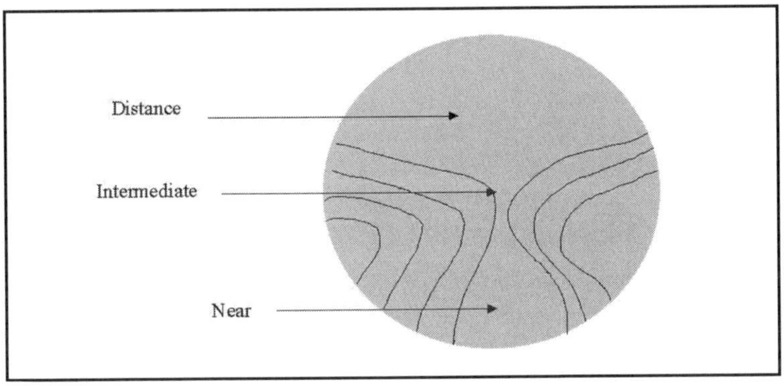

Figure 2-18. A progressive lens consists of three primary zones: distance, intermediate and near.

17). Most often, these lens designs have a bifocal at the top and bottom of the lens (sometimes referred to as a double "D" lens design). However, occupational lenses are also available with a bifocal at the top of the lens and a trifocal segment at the bottom. This is especially beneficial for the mid-to high-plus powered patient with presbyopia who experiences significant problems with viewing intermediate and near objects.

Progressives

Progressive lenses are by far the most technologically advanced multifocal lenses; they are aspheric lenses with no segment lines. These lenses mimic natural vision more closely than any other multifocal design.

Progressive lenses consist of distance, intermediate, and near zones (Figure 2-18).

They cause less of an image jump than lined segments because the power differences between the zones are achieved through slight, gradual changes in power, unlike that of conventionally lined bifocals or trifocals. Progressive lenses are sometimes called bifocals but in actuality perform most like trifocals because they offer an intermediate area.

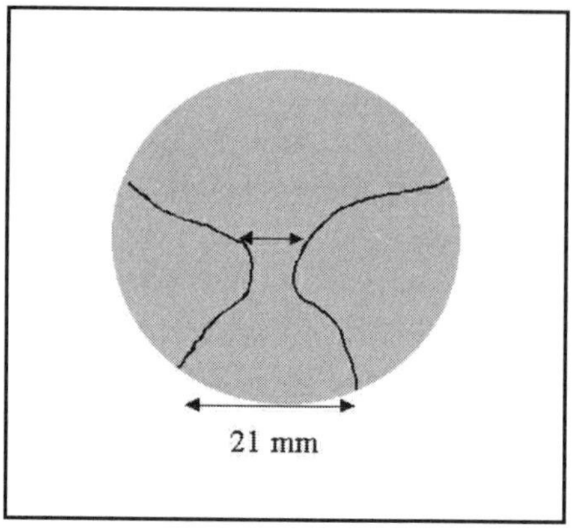

Figure 2-19. Example of a hard design progressive lens.

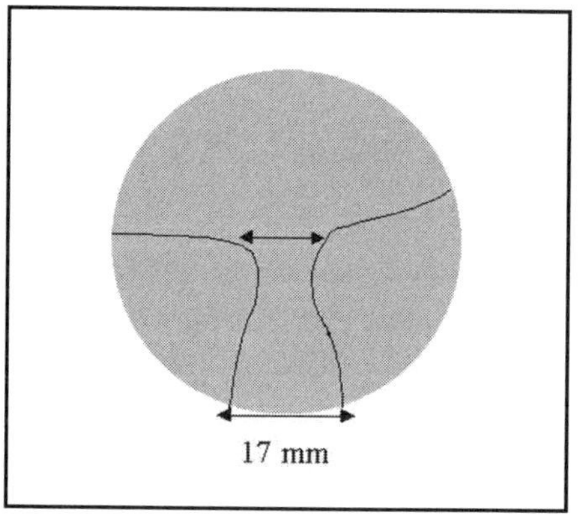

Figure 2-20. Example of a soft design progressive lens.

Manufacturers offer many different progressive designs to meet the visual demands of consumers. Each design performs uniquely depending on the manufacturer and the prescription. There are designs that offer a wide reading area but a more narrow intermediate area. (This would be particularly helpful for patients who require a wide reading field.) These types of progressives are called "hard designs" (Figure 2-19).

A "hard design" progressive offers a vast amount of change over a small area. Unfortunately, hard designs generally produce more peripheral problems (especially if the prescription calls for a significant degree of cylinder correction). Generally, a wider reading area also produces increased peripheral cylinder aberrations that manifest over the 180° line. Aberrations over the 180° line are usually those that prove bothersome to the patient.

A "soft design" is a progressive that has a wide intermediate zone with a more narrow reading area (Figure 2-20). (This would be beneficial for a computer user who can benefit from a wider intermediate field.) A "soft" design has a slight amount of change over a small area. This lens design is called a "soft design" because the smaller reading area results in "softer" (or less noticeable) peripheral cylinder aberrations. Like all progressive lenses, peripheral cylinder aberrations are compounded by high cylinder corrections.

Many progressive lenses are somewhat of a combination of these two designs.

Often times, patients complain of peripheral aberrations that are inherent in all progressive lens designs. The peripheral difficulties are due to unwanted cylinder aberrations created by the design. Unwanted peripheral cylinder power is compounded by additional cylinder in the prescription as well as the power and width of the bifocal. For this reason, patients with high cylin-

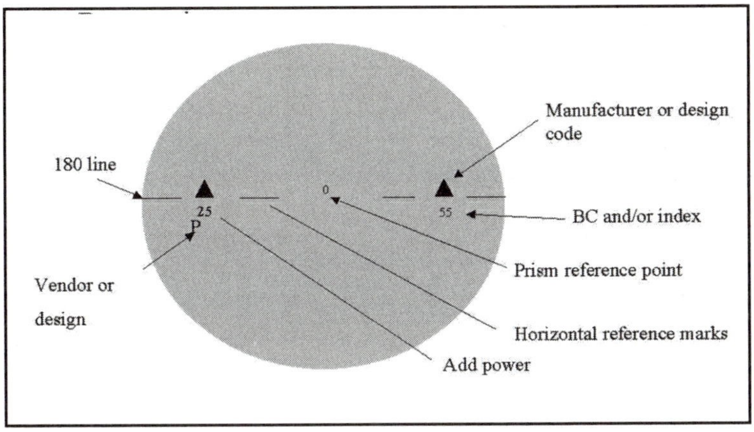

Figure 2-21. Engravings and markings on a progressive lens.

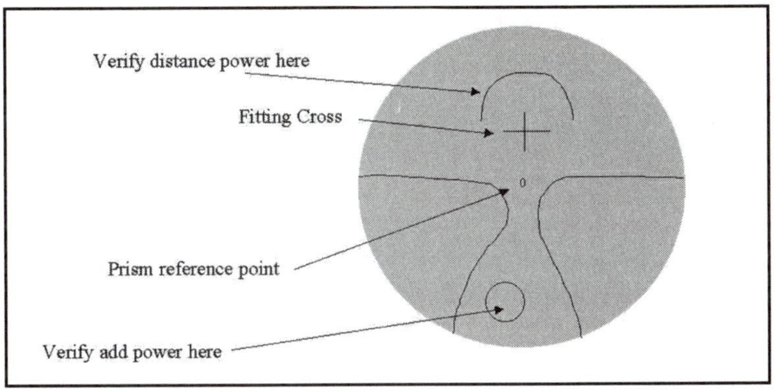

Figure 2-22. Progressive lens with verification markings.

der corrections (over 2.00 D) sometimes have difficulty adjusting to progressive lenses. However, manufacturers are constantly striving to produce more advanced progressive lenses, including lenses that provide better vision for patients with high cylinder corrections. Progressives with toric lens designs have recently been created to address this challenge.

Selecting the most appropriate progressive design is crucial in meeting or exceeding the patient's expectations of the new lenses. Determining the best design is accomplished by becoming educated about the features of the lens designs that are available and by matching these designs with the needs of the wearer.

Progressive lenses have etchings or markings engraved into the front lens surface to indicate the particular lens design as well as the power of the near addition (Figure 2-21). These etchings are more easily viewed when held up to a bright light or if held over steam (as from a tint unit). The markings also include dashes that designate the 180° line (useful to determine if the lens is on axis) and a fitting cross (which indicates the beginning of the segment portion) (Figure 2-22). The fitting cross should be situated at the center of the patient's pupil. Thus it is important to indicate monocular pupillary distance when ordering the lenses to ensure the accurate placement of the optical center and the near segment.

Just above the fitting cross is an arch. It is within this arch that the distance lens power should be verified with the lensometer. Just beneath the fitting cross is a dot representing the location of the optical center or the prism reference point. Each lens is inspected with the lensometer at the dot to verify that the lenses are not vertically unbalanced. The bifocal power should be inspected in the circle present at the bottom of the lenses. The circle is slightly inset and represents the area

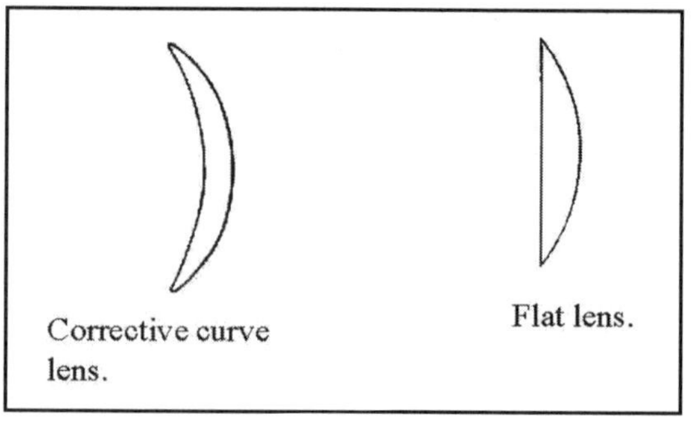

Figure 2-23. Flat and corrective curve lenses.

with the truest add power. As with all multifocal lenses, the truest add power reading for plus lenses is obtained by inspecting the lenses from the front side. (Turn the glasses around and neutralize the distance power and near power from the front side of the lenses. The difference between these two readings is the accurate bifocal power.)

Patients should be informed that their best vision with progressives is achieved through the central corridor of the lenses, both at the point of sale and when the glasses are dispensed. Objects viewed through the periphery of the lenses are generally not quite as clear as objects seen through the central portion.

Special Lens Designs

Corrective Curve Lenses

A lens which could produce the same quality of vision thorough the periphery as through the optical center of the lens would need to have a radius that corresponded with the radius of the moving eyeball. This way, the vertex distance between the cornea and the lens would remain unchanged regardless of the position of the wearer's eye. Such a lens, especially in plus powered corrections, would be very thick and heavy. A lens made to these specifications would be nearly impossible to produce and would not readily mount in modern day frames.[1]

Lenses used in the optical industry today are mathematically designed to improve optical performance in the periphery of the lens. These lenses are called "corrective curve" lenses. Corrective curve lenses, unlike flat lenses that produced significant peripheral problems, couple specific base curves with a given prescription to produce a lens that will have minimal peripheral aberrations (Figure 2-23). Base curve selection charts are available from lens manufacturers and are easily used to determine the most appropriate base curve selection for a given lens power.

Corrective curve lenses enhance the performance of flat lens designs by controlling spherical aberration, chromatic aberration, distortion, and cylindrical aberration. Spherical aberration occurs when a ray of light is not focused to a single point on the retina. Patients experiencing this problem may complain of blurred vision. Chromatic aberration, mentioned earlier, occurs when white light is broken up into its spectral components. Distortion problems caused by a poor base curve selection often results in a "pin cushion" effect (lines appear to curve inward) with strong plus lenses, or a "barrel" effect (lines appear to curve outward) with high minus lenses. Cylinder aberration in the periphery of a lens causes a patient to experience a "swimmy" sensation. The patient may state that images seem wavy or that objects appear to move when viewed through the outer edges of the lenses. (Cylinder aberration problems are, to some degree, inherent in all progressive lens designs.)

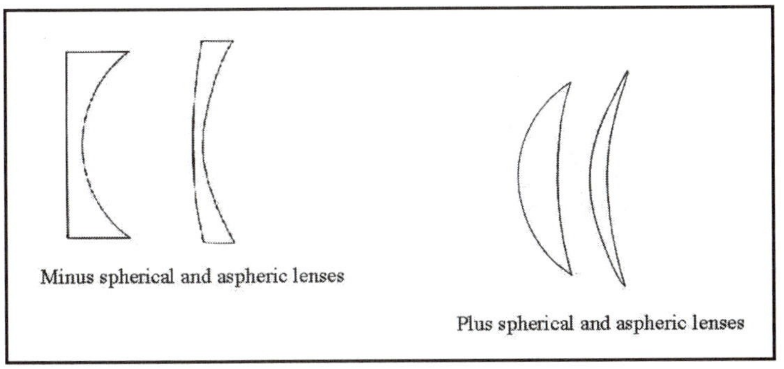

Figure 2-24. Aspheric and spherical lens designs.

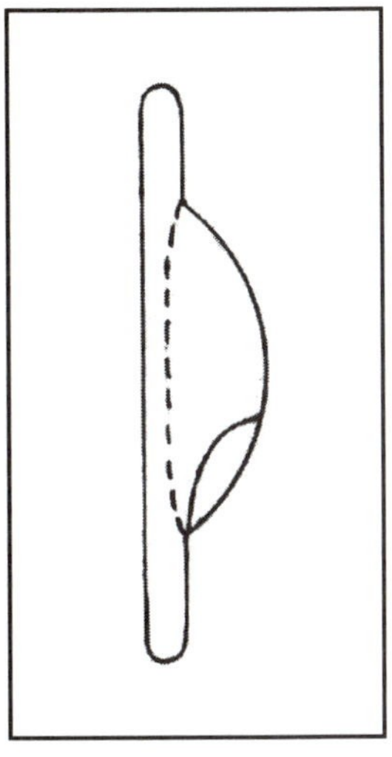

Figure 2-25. Lenticular bowl lens.

Aspherics

Aspheric lenses are mathematically enhanced to produce improved peripheral optics and the cosmetic appearance of the lenses. The curvatures of an aspheric design change in the outer portions of the lens (Figure 2-24). This results in better peripheral vision, a more cosmetically appealing lens, and an increased field of vision. This is especially true with mid- to high-powered lenses. In addition, the size of the patient's eyes appear more normal than with conventional base curves. Aspheric lenses are also flatter and thinner than lenses with spherical curves, and are available in plastic resins (conventional or high index) in a multitude of single vision and multifocal lens styles. Combining aspheric designs with high index materials results in lenses that perform exceptionally well in all areas while also producing a cosmetically pleasing finished product.

Cataract or Aphakic Lenses

Cataract lenses are high plus prescription lenses that are required for individuals who have had their crystalline lens removed (usually due to cataracts).

Cataract lenses are aspheric lenses that are available as lenticular designs (Figure 2-25). This means a minus lenticular carrier (lenticular bowl) is used to house the high powered plus prescription. This type of lens is lighter than a conventional full field aspheric (Figure 2-26); however, it does not offer much peripheral vision. A "Super-Modular" cataract lens is a blended aphakic lens that is lighter than a conventional cataract lens, yet is more cosmetically acceptable than a lenticular lens.

OptA
OphT
LV

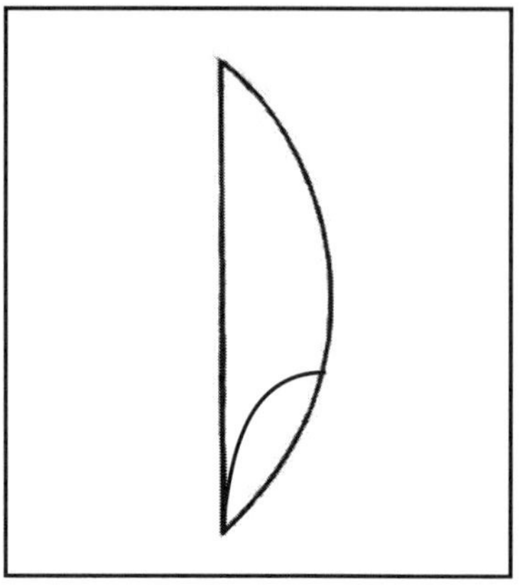

Figure 2-26. Full field aspheric design.

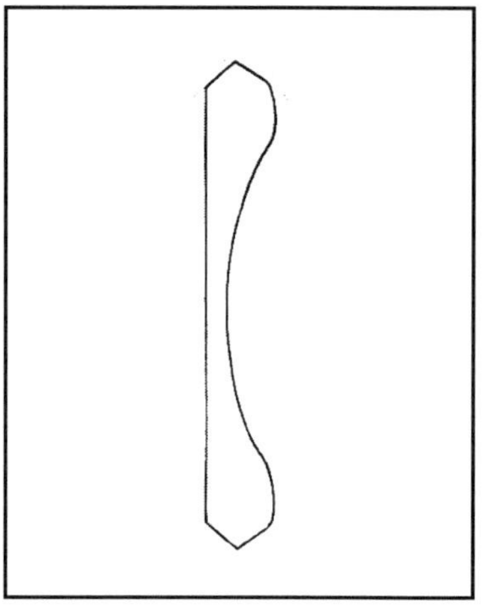

Figure 2-27. Blended myodisc.

Frames selected for cataract lenses should be as small as tolerable to control the weight and thickness of the lenses. They should be fit as close to the eye as possible in order to provide a wide field of vision for the patient.

Lenses for High Myopia

OptA LV

A myodisc or blended myodisc lens is used for patients who have very high myopia. It is a lenticular lens with a carrier, and produces a clear central area for vision with a significantly thinner lens edge (Figure 2-27). The myodisc lens design is generally considered for high minus powers beginning at -12.00 D and is more cosmetically acceptable when compared to conventionally ground high minus lenses. It usually incorporates a plano front curve with a cylinder component (if necessary) and a plano or plus powered carrier with a high minus bowl on the back curve. The major drawback to this lens style is it offers very little peripheral vision. Because of this, patients may complain of "tunnel vision." When selecting a frame style for this lens it is important to choose a sturdy frame with a heavy eyewire and deep lens groove. Many frame manufacturers offer frame styles that are more suitable for high minus lens designs, such as the myodisc; ask your frame representatives.

Another lens for high myopia is the biconcave lens (Figure 2-28). This lens is concave and ground on both the front and back surface, resulting in an overall thinner and lighter-weight lens.

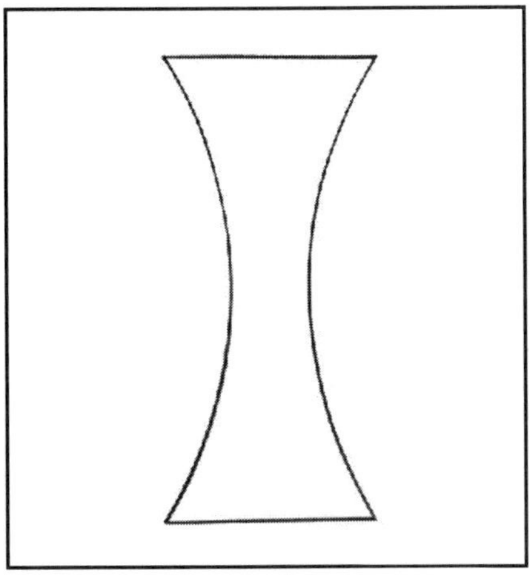

Figure 2-28. Biconcave.

A biconcave or double concave lens is one that has a matching radius of curvature on either side of the lens.

Unfortunately, biconcave designs offer little peripheral vision. The best frame selection for a biconcave design is a sturdy plastic frame or metal style that is specially designed for high minus lenses. Frames with extra long end pieces on the frame front are particularly useful for fitting high minus lenses because they allow the temples to close even though the edges of the lenses are thick.

Safety Lenses

The Occupational Safety and Health Administration (OSHA) is a federal bureau that governs safety eyewear regulations in industrial as well as educational environments. Document ANSI Z87.1-1989, published by the American National Standards Institute, Inc., is a concise composition that thoroughly explains safety eyewear regulations. To assure compliance with these standards, it is recommended that optical establishments dispensing, surfacing, and/or edging safety eyewear be thoroughly informed of the material in the document. The standard for safety eyewear is ANSI Z87.1-1989, and the standard for dress (everyday) eyewear is ANSI Z80.1-1995. Both are available from the Optical Laboratory Association (OLA) by calling (703) 359-2830. OptA OphA OphMT

The safety standard states that ANSI approved safety lenses must have a minimum thickness of 3.0 mm. The exception is lenses of +3.00 D or more, which must have a minimum thickness of 2.5 mm. (The idea here is that plus lenses of this power will have a center thickness that will be at least 2.5 - 3.0 mm which will be thick enough, depending on the lens material as well as the final thickness, to withstand shattering on impact.) The lenses must also have the initials of the laboratory that manufactured them etched into the upper edge of the lenses. (The manufacturer is considered to be the lab that edges the lenses.) The etchings should be in a position that will not interfere with the wearer's vision. Lenses that meet the thickness requirements but do not have the etchings are not considered to be approved safety lenses. (Lens etchings are actually sandblasted into the lenses. This can pose its own problems in a full-service laboratory by creating airborn dust particles that can scratch exposed lenses. It is wise to encase the etching machinery to minimize scratching problems in the laboratory.)

(Special purpose lenses must also have an "S" marked on the lenses to signify that the lenses are for special purposes [Figure 2-29]. An example of special purpose occupational lenses

Figure 2-29. Etched safety lens (special purpose).

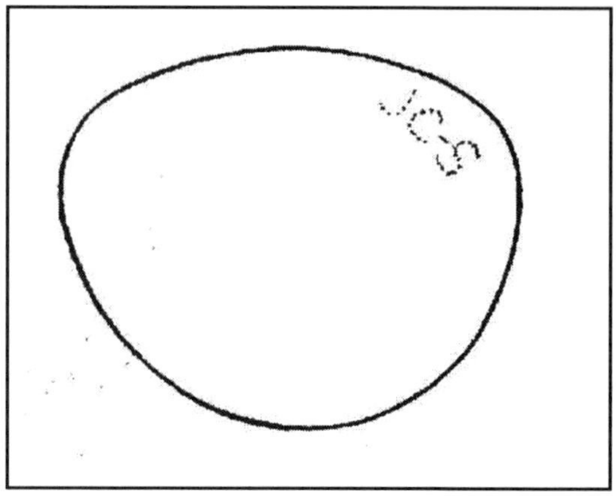

would be those that are needed by welders. Protective lenses for someone in this occupation must have a filter that guards the welder from damaging optical radiation.)

ANSI approved safety lenses are to be mounted only in approved Z-87 frames. ANSI approved frames must have Z87 stamped on the frame front as well as on the temples.

No other combination of frame and lenses denotes ANSI approved safety eyewear. For example, an individual may not mount dress ophthalmic lenses into a safety eyewear frame. Likewise, safety lenses may not be mounted into a dress eyewear frame. Patients may desire a safety frame yet do not want the thicker safety lenses made for the frame, or vice versa, or they may require safety lenses for their occupation but want the lenses mounted into a dress eyewear frame. To be compliant with the standard, as well as providing maximum protection for the patient, neither choice is available.

Any material can be used for safety lenses; however, polycarbonate is the safest lens material on the market and is virtually shatterproof when the thickness rules for safety eyewear are followed. For safety reasons, individuals working in hazardous situations or occupations should be advised of the benefits of polycarbonate lenses, which will be discussed in more detail later in this chapter.

Slab-Off Prism

OphT

Single vision or multifocal patients who are anisometropic (have unequal refractive powers in the two eyes, particularly when one eye requires a plus correction and the other eye requires a minus correction) often need glasses with a specially ground lens treatment called *slab-off*. The unbalanced refractive powers of the two lenses, especially if the difference between the two corrections is greater than 1.50 D, cause prismatic problems at near. Because of this, the patient is not able to achieve binocular vision (or one fused image) when reading with the glasses. A slab-off lens remedies this problem by correcting for vertical prism imbalances.

A lens with slab-off treatment has a fine, raised horizontal line across the lens. If the lens is a bifocal, the line appears equal with the segment line (Figure 2-30). Most often it is barely visible and does not pose cosmetic problems.

Specialty labs add slab-off prismatic treatments to lenses either using bicentric grinding methods or molded resins. Some lens manufacturers offer semi-finished lens blanks with slab-off treatments of varying prismatic degrees that are pre-cast on the front surface of the lenses.

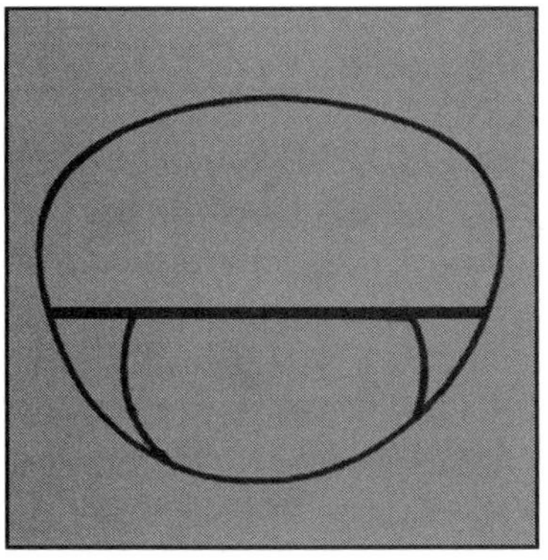

Figure 2-30. Slab-off prism.

Lens Materials

OptA OphA

Lens styles and designs are available in many different materials. For example, a specific progressive lens might be manufactured in CR-39, high index, polycarbonate, and glass. Check your lens availability guides to determine designs and materials.

CR-39

CR-39 is regular plastic resin and the most common lens material used today. Created by chemists at Columbia Southern Corporation in 1942, "CR" stands for Columbia Resin and "39" indicates that the 39th test resin produced by the company was successful. It is a "lab friendly" material that is lightweight and very stable. It is less likely to shatter than glass. CR-39 doesn't easily scratch during the manufacturing process (especially if a factory scratch resistant coating is applied) and it readily accepts tints and coatings. CR-39 is available in most all lens styles including single vision, bifocals, and multifocals.

Glass

Glass lenses are available in a variety of glass materials including flint glass (or lead glass, which is a high index material), crown glass, and barium crown glass (also high index, used in multifocal glass segments). Glass lenses are heat or chemically tempered to resist shattering.

Air or heat tempering is accomplished by placing glass lenses into a thermal heating unit and heating the lenses for a specified time (depending on the size and weight of the lenses). After heating, the lenses are slowly cooled. This heating and cooling process results in glass lenses that are more resistant to shattering.

Chemical tempering of glass lenses is done by placing the lenses into a treatment unit over night. The chemicals used and length of time needed to accomplish this process are determined by the glass material (photochromic materials require different chemicals than clear glass) and the prescription. Labs often choose to chemically treat glass lenses (rather than heat treating them) if the lenses are of a very high power or if they are of a complex nature (executive bifocals, slab-off designs, etc).

With an Abbe value of 59, crown glass refracts light more purely than any other lens material. However, the lenses are heavy and pose a safety risk, particularly for children and those in some occupations.

LV

Photochromic glass, or PhotoGray (Corning Glass Co, Corning, NY.), was developed in the 1960's and experienced incredible popularity in the 70's and 80's. It is still dispensed today. PhotoGray lenses change from light inside to dark outside. Silver halide is used in the manufacturing process of these glass lenses; it darkens in color depending on the degree of ultraviolet (UV) rays striking the lens surface. Thus, it will turn dark even on a cloudy day, since UV rays still emit through the clouds.

LV

Transitions

Transitions (Pittsburgh Plate Glass Industries, Pittsburgh, PA) is a photochromatic or phototropic material that is infused into the front surface of a resin lens. The material darkens and lightens depending on the amount of ultraviolet light that strikes the front lens surface. Transitions lenses are immensely popular today and are available from many lens manufacturers. Lenses with this photochromatic material, depending on the vendor, are available in several different colors. Brown, gray, and even a darker version are available to the industry. Consult your wholesale laboratory or lens vendors for more information regarding these lenses. Photochromic (phototropic) safety lenses must have a "V" etched into the lenses indicating that they are of varying tint.

High-Index Lenses

High index lenses are made of denser materials than more conventional materials such as CR-39. Because the material is denser, it takes less of the high index material to refract light in the same way as conventional materials, thus the lens is thinner and lighter. High index materials are available in plastic resins and glass. They are also available in a wide variety of indices, from a medium index, such as 1.537, to a very high index of 1.66.

When selling or working with high index materials is it important to know if the lenses are decentered or laid out "on center." If the lenses are "on center" it is necessary to keep the frame size to a minimum to guarantee that the job will cut out after decentering the lenses. (However, it is always beneficial to select smaller frames when it comes to lenses with higher powers.) Choosing an appropriate frame size results in thinner, lighter lenses.

Maximizing the overall appearance of high index lenses is obtained by controlling either the center thickness of minus lenses or the edge thickness of plus lenses. Patients will realize the full benefits of high index lenses if the lenses are ground as thin as possible, based on the recommendations of the manufacturer.

Polycarbonate

Polycarbonate was introduced to the optical industry in the 1970's and is the lens of choice when safety is an issue. It is extremely lightweight and, due to its high refractive index, produces thinner lenses than conventional materials.

Because of its impact-absorbing ability, it is very soft in nature. Caution is needed when handling polycarbonate in the lab to avoid scratching. Also, acetone cannot be used on this material, as it will split the surface of a lens. Tinting and neutralizing polycarbonite lenses should be done with dye pots at a lower temperature than standard to avoid crazing or splitting the lens surface. Polycarbonate is difficult to roll and polish due to its waxy nature. Rather than hand polishing the edge, some laboratories use liquid edge polish or dressing to achieve a shiny edge finish.

The Abbe value for polycarbonate is 31. Because of this, some patients (especially in the higher minus powers) may complain of peripheral chromatic aberration problems with this material. Chromatic problems with polycarbonate (or any other ultra-high refractive index material such as 1.66) can be minimized if:

1. the optical centers of the lenses are specified and ground into the correct position
2. the monocular PD is correct (for single vision and progressive styles only)
3. the frame size is kept to a minimum

Reference

1. Stein HA, Slatt BJ, Stein RM. *The Ophthalmic Assistant: Fundamentals and Clinical Practice.* St. Louis, Mo: The C.V. Mosby Company; 1988.

Chapter 3

Instrumentation and Measurements

KEY POINTS

- The lensometer is used to determine the spherical power, cylinder power and axis, and optical center of a lens. It is also used to determine the degree and direction of prism.
- Pupillary distance, or PD, is used to ensure that the optical center of the lens is ground to coincide with the patient's visual axis.
- The vertex distance (VD) is the distance (in millimeters) between the back surface of an ophthalmic lens and the patient's cornea. A distometer is a calibration tool that is used to determine this measurement.
- It is essential to take accurate measurements of the spectacle frame each time an order is placed. The "A" measurement refers to the eye size of the frame. The "B" measurement is the vertical measurement. The "ED" is the effective diameter of a lens. The DBL (distance between lenses) is the width of the bridge.
- The minimum blank size is determined by adding the "ED" measurement with the total amount of decentration plus 2 mm for edging purposes.
- The segment height determines the placement of a multifocal segment. It is given in millimeters and is measured from the deepest portion of the eyewire.
- It is necessary to specify the optical center placement for single vision lenses of substantial power, or when using lens materials with a high refractive index.
- The lens clock, also known as the Geneva lens measure, is an instrument used to determine the base curve of an ophthalmic lens.

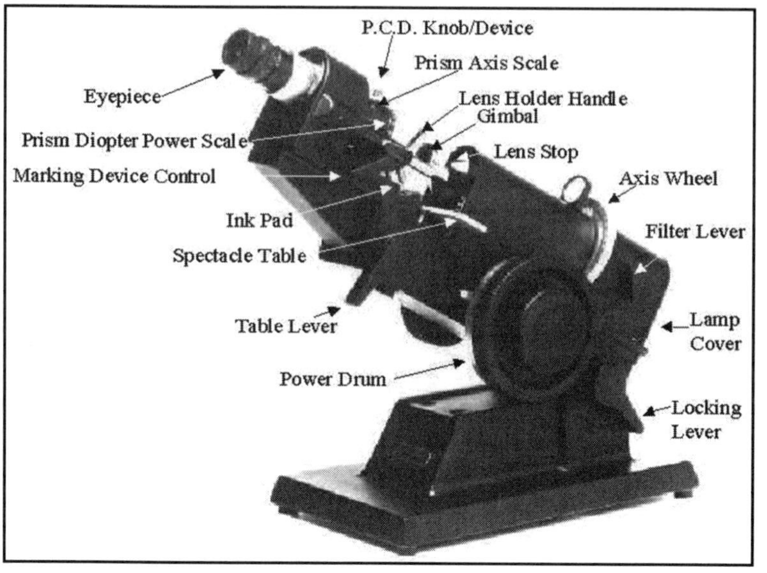

Figure 3-1. Manual lensometer.

OptA OphA CL

Lensometry

The manual lensometer is the most frequently used piece of equipment in the optical dispensary (Figure 3-1). With it, one can neutralize or read the power of an ophthalmic lens or contact lens. It is used to determine the spherical power, cylinder power and axis, and optical center of a lens. It is also used to determine the degree and direction of prism. While there are several automated lensometers on the market, these machines often give false power readings or mistakenly report the amount of prism ground into a lens (especially when neutralizing progressive lenses). For this reason, opticians and technicians need good manual lensometry skills.

A manual lensometer is an intricate piece of machinery; skillful operation of this essential piece of equipment is achieved only through routine usage. The most common method is described here; readers are encouraged to consult the user's manual of their particular instrument.

Instrument Set Up

Step One

Focus the eyepiece. Before attempting to neutralize lenses, it is important to focus the eyepiece (Figure 3-2). The eyepiece is actually a series of lenses that are part of the lensometer. To focus the eyepiece, first turn the power drum to plano (or 0 power), then turn the eyepiece to its most plus position. Without inserting lenses or a pair of spectacles into the lensometer, inspect the reticle (Figure 3-3) through the eyepiece. (The reticle is the image of circles and numbers that is used to locate the optical center of an ophthalmic lens. It is also used to determine prismatic degree and placement.) While viewing the reticle, adjust the eyepiece by turning it slowly toward minus until the numbers and circles appear sharp and focused. Stop as soon as the reticle is clear and go no further. If you continue toward more minus at this point, you will stimulate your accommodation. This could render the reading inaccurate.

If you are working in a large clinic where many people use the same instrument, it is sometimes beneficial to mark your lensometer to avoid repeating these focusing procedures each time a pair of glasses is inspected. Simply focus the eyepiece for yourself and place a mark on the eye-

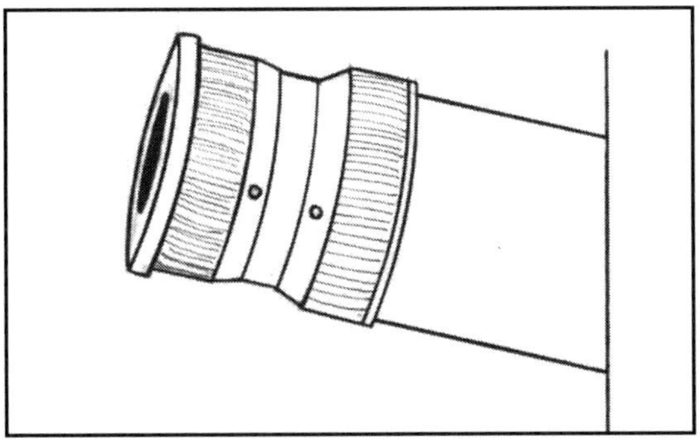

Figure 3-2. Eyepiece.

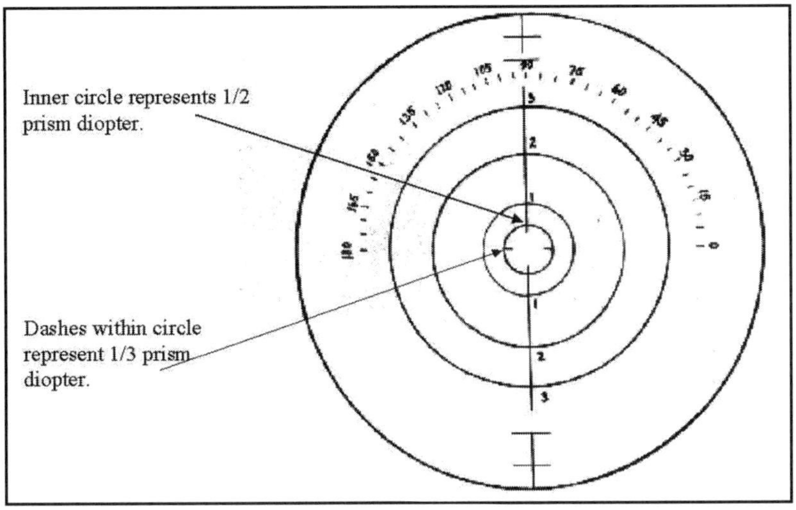

Figure 3-3. Reticle.

piece with a colored grease pencil or marker at the indicator dot to signify your personal adjustment. After doing this, you can quickly turn to your mark on the eyepiece before neutralizing a pair of spectacles.

Step Two

Position the frame on the carriage making sure that both eyewires are evenly placed on the carriage (Figure 3-4). If one eyewire is slightly off the carriage or one of the temples is on top of the power drum, this can significantly alter the reading of the lens power. Likewise, this can also produce a false axis reading.

Step Three

Locate the optical center of the lens by finding the central point at which the cross hairs meet (Figure 3-5). When the optical center of the lens has been located, lock the lens into place with the lens holder. The optical center is the point of an ophthalmic lens where the lens has no prismatic effect on in-coming light. It is not necessarily the geometric center of the lens. When neutralizing a pair of spectacles, it is important to begin with the strongest lens first to ensure correct placement of the optical centers for each lens. (This is very important when dealing with prism, which is covered later.)

After locating the optical center of the strongest lens, lock the lens into place by using the lens holder (Figure 3-6). The lens holder is a device on the lensometer that clamps down on the lens,

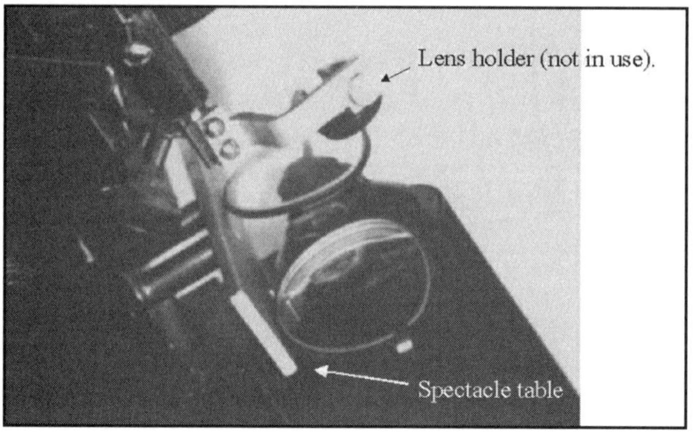

Figure 3-4. Place the eyewires evenly on the spectacle table.

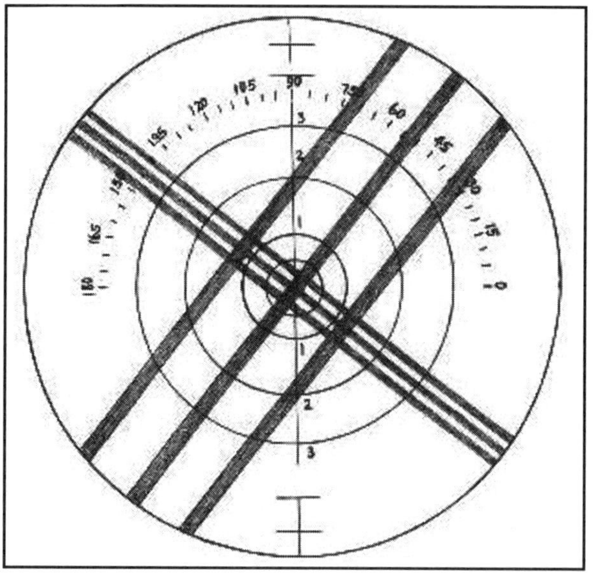

Figure 3-5. The optical center is the central point at which the cross-hairs meet.

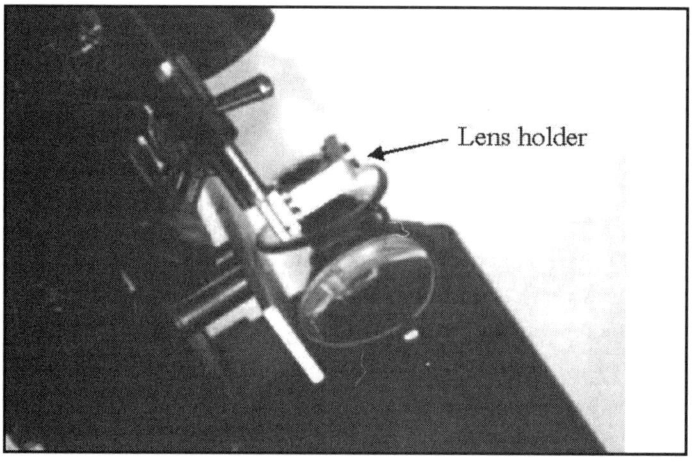

Figure 3-6. Use the lens holder to lock the lens into place.

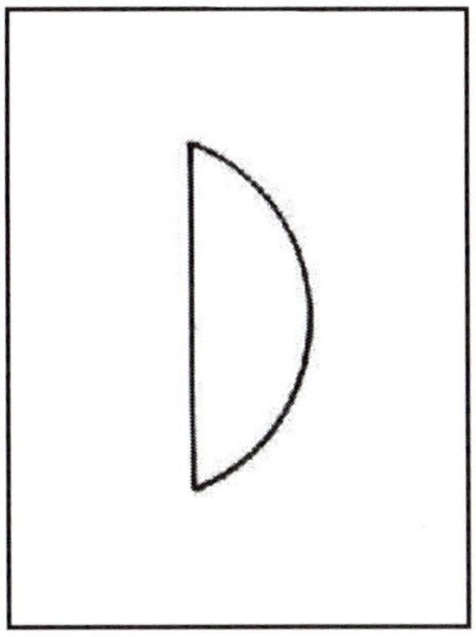

Figure 3-7. Plus spherical lens.

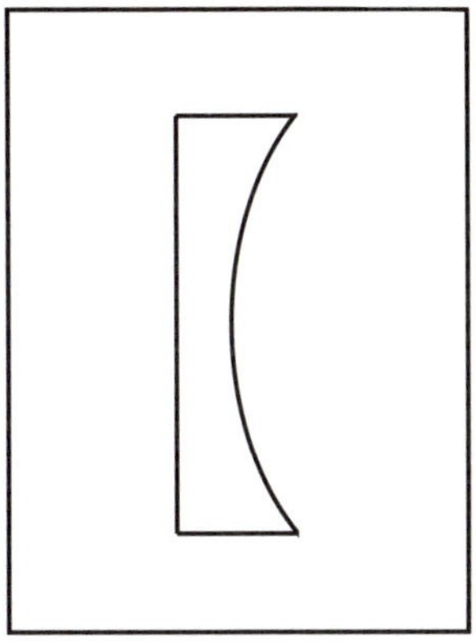

Figure 3-8. Minus spherical lens.

holding it firmly in place. It is important to use this device when obtaining the power of a lens to ensure the accuracy of the neutralization. Use caution when clamping a lens into place. Some materials, such as the new ultra-high refractive index lenses and polycarbonate lenses, are soft and thus easy to scratch. Because of this, lenses are often damaged in the laboratory during the final inspection stage before being dispensed to the patient. Examine the lens holder on your lensometer for damage and take notice of the circular pad that is affixed to the clamp. Is it in good condition? Sometimes this rubber pad will dry out and cause scratches on lenses made of soft materials.

Neutralizing Spectacle Lenses

Spherical lenses are lenses that bring light to a single focus on the retina. This type of a lens consists of the same refractive power in all meridians. A plus spherical lens (Figure 3-7) is convex and appears to have been sliced from a globe. A minus spherical lens (Figure 3-8) is concave and appears to have been cast from the side of a sphere. (For more on lenses and optics, see the Basic Bookshelf title *Optics, Retinoscopy, and Refractometry.*)

Spherocylindrical or compound lenses (Figure 3-9) are necessary for patients who have astigmatism. Instead of being shaped like a sphere, which is perfectly round, an astigmatic eye is not round. It is an irregular shape, somewhat like a football, which produces blurred vision. Thus, astigmatic patients require two separate curvatures to correct their refractive error: a spherical power and a cylindrical power. The cylindrical component of the prescription is ground in the opposite meridian of the patient's visual defect. Grinding the cylinder power in the opposite

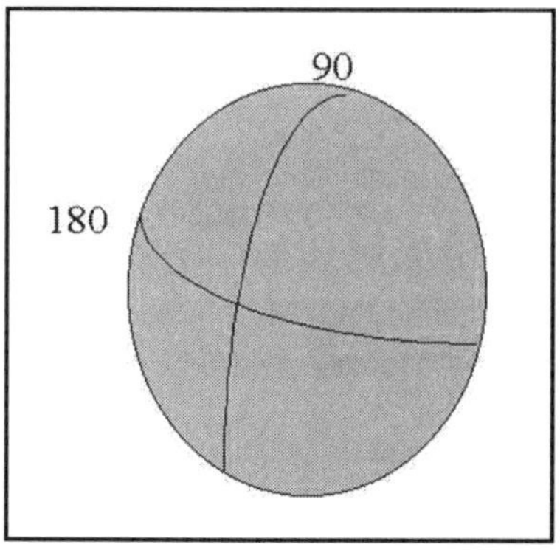

Figure 3-9. Cylindrical lens.

meridian neutralizes the astigmatism. Prescriptions for cylindrical lenses will always include an axis indicating the direction of the cylinder.

Determining if a Lens Is Spherical or Compound

While looking through the eyepiece of a manual lensometer, turn the power drum until you obtain a clear image of the mires. Next, rotate the axis wheel while continuing to inspect the mires through the eyepiece. Do the lines change when you turn the axis wheel? Do they become broken, then come into sharp focus, then seem broken again as you continue to change from one axis to the next? If so, you are inspecting a compound or spherocylindrical lens. Lines or mires that change dramatically as you rotate the axis wheel indicate that the degree of cylindrical power will be significant. Minute changes in the integrity of the mires imply a slight degree of cylinder power.

When viewing a spherical lens with a lensometer, you will notice that the appearance of the mires remains constant. Because a spherical lens is the same power in all meridians, the image of the mires remains unchanged regardless of the position of the axis wheel.

Marking and Measuring the Optical Center

After aligning the optical center of each lens in the middle of the reticle, use the marking device on the lensometer to mark the optical center. The marking device will place three dots of ink on each lens. The center dot is the optical center. Measure from the center dot of one lens to the center dot of the other with a millimeter ruler. This measurement (DBC, or the distance between centers) should match the patient's distance pupillary measurement or be within the ANSI guidelines. If the measurement is not within ANSI standards, the lenses are considered to have induced prism and Prentice's rule (explained later) should be used to calculate the degree of unwanted prism.

Neutralizing a Spherical Lens

1. Adjust the frame on the carriage until the optical center of the strongest lens is well-centered when viewed through the eyepiece.
2. Turn the power drum until the mires are clear and sharp. You should see no alterations in the appearance of the mires; all of the lines should look identical (Figure 3-10). Rotate the axis wheel while viewing the mires through the eyepiece to ensure that the lens is spherical.
3. If needed, sharpen the image of the mires by turning the power drum while looking through the eyepiece. When the mires appear focused and clear, determine the diopter power of the lens

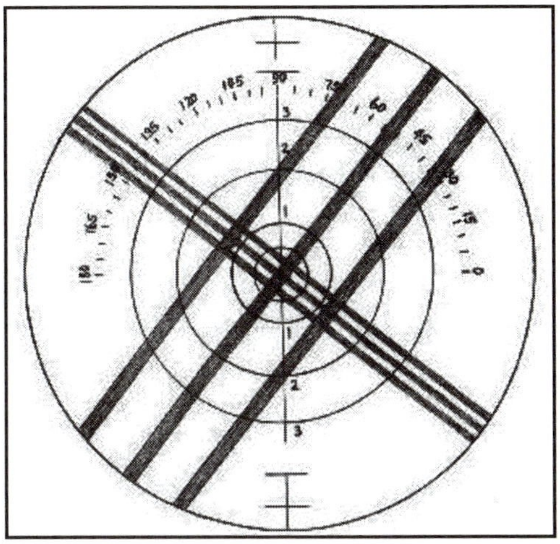

Figure 3-10. Spherical lens viewed through the reticle. Turning the axis wheel results in no alterations in the appearance of the lines.

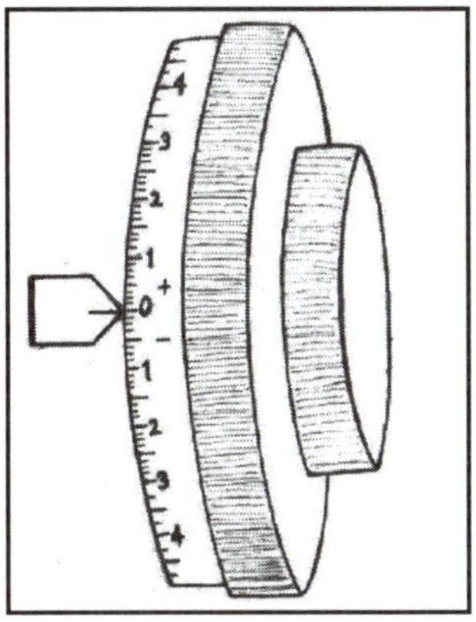

Figure 3-11. The power drum indicating a plano reading.

by inspecting the position of the power wheel (Figure 3-11). Take note of the numerical reading on the power wheel; this is the spherical power of the lens.

Neutralizing a Spherocylindrical Lens

1. Place the frame on the carriage and position the glasses with the optical center of the strongest lens in the center of the reticle.

2. Rotate the power drum *away* from you until the cylinder lines, which are usually the thickest lines, come in clearly. If the cylinder lines only come in clearly when you rotate the power wheel *toward* you, you must then turn the axis wheel until the mires come in clearly when you rotate the power drum away from you. This will be a 90 degree change in axis. You have obtained the minus cylinder correction when the thickest lines are sharp and unbroken. Once this occurs, note the power on the power drum. If the cylinder lines are not perfectly straight, turn the axis wheel until they become very crisp and intact. *Note:* In the optical shop, lenses are always neutralized in minus cylinder. This means that it is necessary to turn the power drum *away* from you when obtaining the cylinder correction of a lens. (Conversely, when neutralizing the lens in plus cylinder, you must turn the power wheel *toward* you.) Turn the axis wheel until the sphere lines, which are the thinnest lines on most lensometers, are unbroken. Then turn the power drum until the lines focus clearly. Note the power indicated on the power drum; this is the spherical power of the lens.

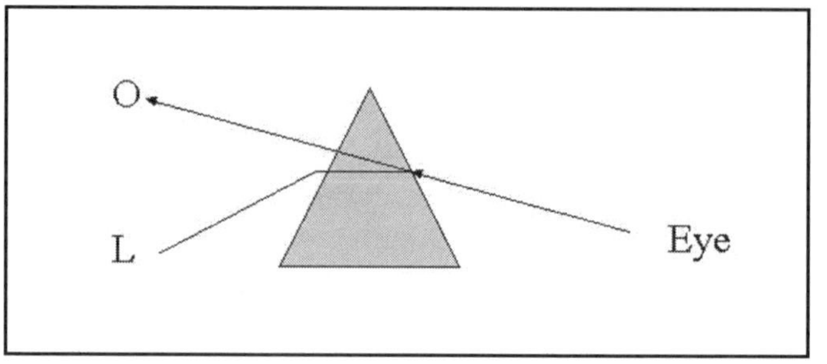

Figure 3-12. If an object is 1 m away, a 1 diopter prism will displace the object's image by 1 cm.

3. Determine the cylinder power of the lenses. The cylinder power is the *difference* between the spherical reading and the cylinder reading on the power drum. (It may help to think of the power drum as a number line.) For example, after neutralizing a lens it is determined that the sphere power is -2.00. After turning the power drum away from you, the cylinder lines come in sharp and clear at a reading of -6.00. The difference between -2.00 and -6.00 is -4.00. Thus the cylinder power of the lens is -4.00.

4. To complete the neutralization of the lens, it is necessary to know the point at which the sphere and cylinder powers meet. In the above example, suppose that the axis wheel reads 090. Thus, the entire neutralization of this lens would be: -2.00 -4.00 x 090.

Determining the Add Power of a Lens

1. Take the distance reading of the lens.

2. Move the lens up slightly so that the bifocal portion of the lens is resting on the lens stop. Clamp the lens down using the lens holder, and rotate the power drum until the sphere lines come in clearly. Note the spherical reading.

3. Now calculate the difference between the bifocal spherical power and the distance spherical power. This is the add power. Example: the distance spherical power reads -2.00 and the bifocal spherical power reads +0.50. The actual add power is +2.50, or (+0.50)-(-2.00) = +2.50.

Note: When reading the bifocal power of a high plus lens (distance power is over +3.00), turn the glasses so that they are facing you and read the front vertex power of the lens. Then move the lens up slightly and read the bifocal power. Subtract the distance reading from the near reading (as above) to determine the true add power. Determining the add power of a high plus lens by neutralizing the back curve will result in a higher, inaccurate reading due to the base curvature of the lens.

Prism

Prismatic correction is often necessary for patients who experience visual problems because of strabismus. (Strabismus is a condition in which the eyes cannot focus together due to eye muscle imbalances. This sometimes results in blurred or double vision.) A prescription for prismatic correction will include the "Δ" sign, indicating that prism is needed. The direction for the base of the prism is indicated by writing BD (base down), BO (base out), BU (base up), and BI (base in). One prism diopter visually displaces an object by 1 cm if the object is 1 m away (Figure 3-12). Stronger prismatic corrections will result in a greater degree of image displacement. The correct amount of prism will create enough visual displacement to enable the patient to appreciate a single, fused image.

Tolerances on prism reference point location and prismatic power.

Prismatic power (Δ)	Tolerance (Δ)
0.00 up to 2.00	±0.25
over 2.00 up to 10.00	±0.37
over 10.00	±0.50

Figure 3-13. ANSI Z80.1-1995 guidelines for prism.

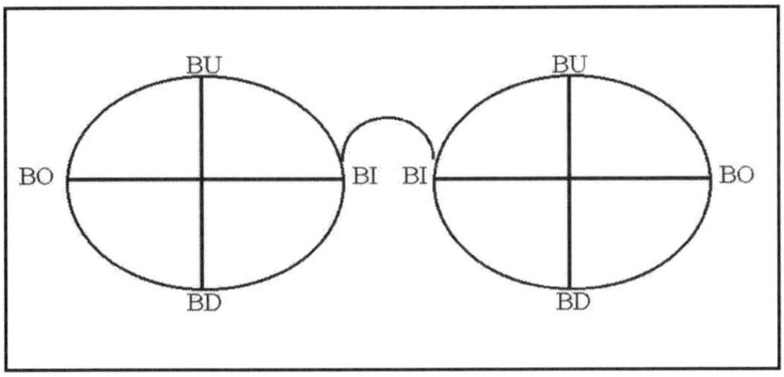

Figure 3-14. Determining prism direction.

It is important to be able to verify prescribed as well as unwanted prism with a manual lensometer. Prism can be incorporated into a lens in two ways: ground-in or induced. Ground-in prism is fabricated directly into the lens when it is made. Induced prism is created by moving the optical center away from the patient's visual axis. Often we think of induced prism as being an error; however, if a patient needs prism correction, it may be produced by grinding it in *or* by decentration. If prism is not ordered and the lenses are decentered, then the induced prism is certainly unwanted and may cause problems for the patient.

Prescribed prism should be verified for accuracy before dispensing, and likewise unwanted prism should be calculated to determine if the lens is to be rejected or dispensed to the patient. A slight degree of unwanted prism, based on the power of the lens, is regarded as tolerable by ANSI standards (Figure 3-13).

Determining Prism with the Lensometer

The direction of a prism is determined by its base. The reticle is divided into four quadrants (Figure 3-14). To calculate the direction of the prism, it is important to know in which quadrant the optical center appears, as well as its relationship to the bridge of the frame.

Verifying Ground-In Prism

1. Inspect the written optical invoice or chart to verify the amount and direction of the prescribed prism in a pair of spectacles.

2. Begin inspecting the glasses by placing the frame on the lensometer carriage making sure that both eyewires are in an even position on the carriage.

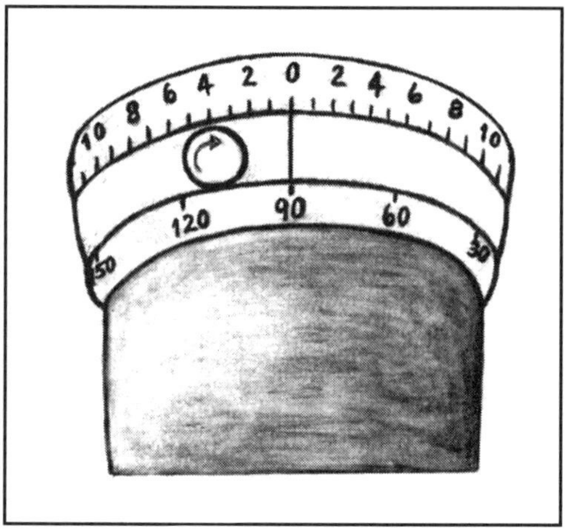

Figure 3-15. Prism compensating device.

3. View the optical center of the right lens through the eyepiece. Notice how the optical center corresponds with the markings on the reticle. (The rings on the reticle are numbered to determine the degree of prism diopter.) For example, if this lens should have 2 diopters of prism in the right lens, then the optical center of this lens would coincide with the #2 ring on the reticle.

4. Figure the prism direction by checking the relationship of the frame bridge to the optical center. If the optical center is ground nasally on the 180 degree line, then the direction of the base is BI. (This would be BI because the nasal area of the face is the most inward position of the lens, see Figure 3-14.) If the optical center were instead ground in the temporal position, it would be BO because this would be the most outward position of the lens.

5. Mark the lenses with the marking device and measure the PD on the glasses; this should coincide with the PD indicated on the job order.

6. If needed, calculate the prism ground into the left lens by repeating these same steps. *Do not alter the position of the frame carriage when moving the left lens into position on the lens stop.*

Verifying Prism Diopters Over 5.00 D

Use the prism compensating device (PCD) (Figure 3-15) to inspect lenses with a high degree of prism correction. The PCD is located close to the eyepiece of the lensometer and moves horizontally to determine horizontal prism (BI or BO), or can be locked in the vertical position to verify lenses with vertical prism (BU or BD). It is important to first move the device into the appropriate position before inspecting prism lenses. When verifying lenses with horizontal prism, the device should be locked into the 180 degree position. Lock the device into the 90 degree position to inspect lenses with vertical prism.

First, position the strongest lens on the lens stop. Move the frame carriage to hold the lens firmly in place. While looking at the reticle through the eyepiece, rotate the silver knob on the PCD until the optical center of the lens is centered in the reticle.

The prism scale on the device indicates the degree of prism present in the lens. The prism direction is determined by the position of the device as well as the position of the bridge of the frame.

Repeat the steps for the other lens. Mark the lenses with the marking device to ensure that the pupillary measurement is accurate.

Most lensometers are capable of neutralizing up to 20.00 D of prism power with the PCD. The total power of the prism scale accounts for 15.00 D of prism and the reticle accounts for 5.00

D. To verify prism over 15.00 D, move the lensometer's optical center by 5.00 D by turning the silver knob on the device. This allows for an additional 5.00 D when reading a lens with a great amount of prism. For example, if verifying a lens with 20.00 D BO prism, move the optical center of the lensometer in 5.00 D and then use the PCD. The prism scale would tell us that the prism power is 15.00 D BO, which would give us a total of 20.00 D (because we already accounted for the other 5.00 D by moving the optical center of the lensometer). To put it mathematically: 15.00 D – (-5.00 D) = 20.00 D.

It is worth mentioning that you should always set the PCD back to zero after each use. If this is not done, the next person to use the lensometer will either be unable to find the mires (if they are shifted off of the lensometer reticle totally) or will "find" prism in the lenses. A corollary is to check the PCD yourself before neutralizing a pair of lenses to avoid being fooled.

OphMT

Verifying Induced Prism

Ground-in prism generally cannot be moved to another position on the reticle (ie, 2 BI cannot be made to read 4 BO). However, induced prism often can be centered and/or moved to different positions on the reticle. This type of prism should be calculated after first aligning the optical center in the middle of the reticle. Then use Prentice's rule (below) to determine the amount of induced prism depending on the power of the lenses.

Prentice's Rule

Prentice's rule is a formula that is used to figure the amount of induced prism in a lens. Lenses with inaccurate pupillary measurements, unevenly ground optical centers, or purposefully decentered lenses for strabismus result in prism. It is especially important to be able to determine the degree of unprescribed prism because the ANSI standard for spectacle lenses allows for only a slight degree of unwanted prism.

The tolerable degree of unwanted prism is determined by the dioptric power of the prescription. Decentered high-powered lenses produce more unwanted prism than lower powered lenses. Likewise, high-powered lenses that meet the ANSI standards must be closely ground to exact requirements in order to pass these specifications.

Prentice's rule: P = hD

P = prism diopters

h = centimeters from the optical center

D= diopters of power

Example: A +4.00 D lens should have the pupillary measurement ground at 31 mm. However, an error has been made and the measurement was ground at 36 mm (a difference of 5 mm). To calculate the amount of unwanted prism induced by this lens:

Our formula is: P= (0.5)*(4.00)

(*Note:* Change mm to cm by moving the decimal point one space to the left, thus 5 mm becomes 0.5 cm.)

The answer is 2.00 BO, which is greater than the tolerable value per the ANSI standard for this lens power.

Direction of Induced Prism

After calculating the degree of induced prism, it is then necessary to determine the direction of the prism.

Plus lenses are "against motion" convergent lenses. This means that if you were to move a plus lens while viewing it through the lensometer, you would see the mires shift in the opposite direction of your movement.

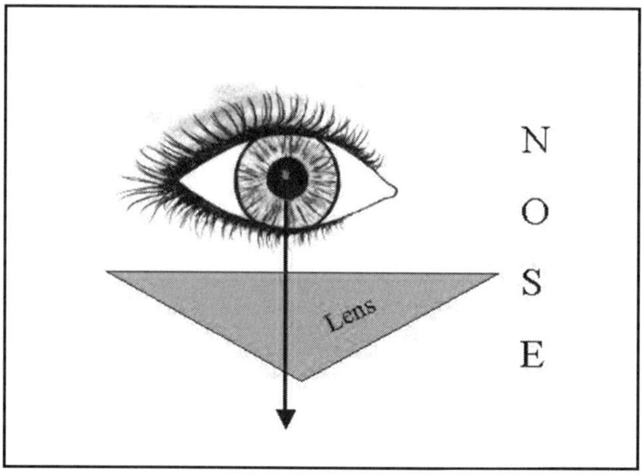

Figure 3-16. A plus lens ground with a narrow OC placement results in BI prism

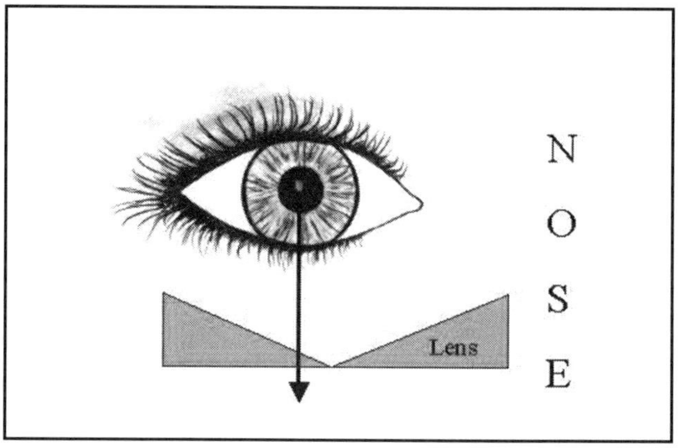

Figure 3-17. A minus lens ground with a narrow OC placement results in BO prism

Minus lenses are "with motion" divergent lenses. This means that if you were to move a minus lens while inspecting it with a lensometer, you would see the mires relocate in the same direction as your movement. Understanding this information about movement is necessary to determine the direction of induced prism in a lens.

Optical centers ground on the optical axis have no prismatic effect for plus or minus lenses. However, a plus lens that has been ground with a narrow optical center placement (ie, the optical centers are moved inward, or the DBC is narrower than the patient's PD)creates BI prism (Figure 3-16). A minus lens that has been ground with a narrow optical center creates BO prism (Figure 3-17). When determining the direction of the prism, it may be helpful to remember that lenses are really prisms connected either base to base (plus lenses) or apex to apex (minus lenses). If this concept seems confusing, it is sometimes useful to actually draw the situation on paper to assess the placement of the optical center and the resultant direction of the induced prism.

OptA
OphA

Pupillary Distance

Before ordering lenses for a patient it is necessary to take a measurement of the patient's PD in millimeters. (Some also refer to this as the interpupillary distance, or IPD.) This is to ensure that the optical center of the lens is ground to coincide with the patient's visual axis.

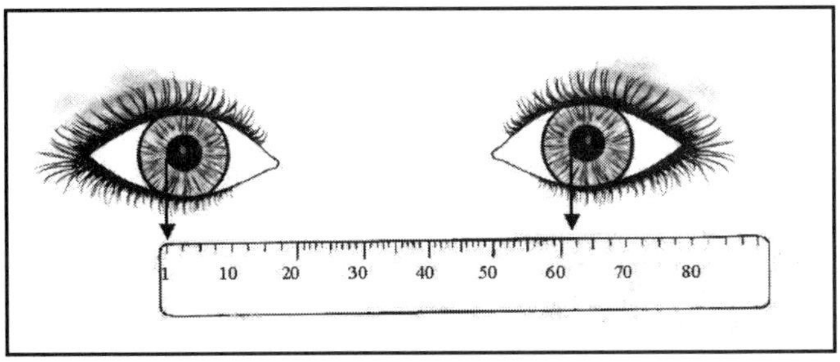

Figure 3-18. Determining the binocular pupillary measurement with a millimeter ruler.

Sometimes the PD is needed as a binocular measurement (both eyes) and other times as a monocular measurement (each eye independently). Monocular measurements are needed when ordering progressive lenses or when ordering lenses with a high refractive index, such as polycarbonate or high index. By specifying the monocular optical center of each lens, you are ensuring that your patient receives optimum vision with the new lenses.

Both of these measurements can be obtained by using a millimeter ruler or corneal reflection pupillometer (CRP). Using a CRP is by far the most accurate means of obtaining the pupillary measurement.

Measuring the Pupillary Distance with a Millimeter Ruler

Method 1: Binocular Pupillary Measurement

Position yourself directly in front of the patient. Place the millimeter ruler on the patient's bridge and close your right eye. Ask the patient to look directly at your open eye. Now align the 0 on the ruler with the *outside* edge of the pupil of the patient's right eye. Without moving the ruler, close your left eye and open your right eye. Note the number on the ruler at the *inside* edge of the pupil of the patient's left eye. This reading is the binocular distance (in millimeters) between the patient's pupils (Figure 3-18). This method measures the outside edge of the left pupil to the inside edge of the right pupil. (Measuring from the outside to the inside edge of each pupil is easier than trying to calculate the center of each pupil, and the resulting dimension is the same.) This method is inappropriate if the patient's pupils have been dilated.

Method 2: Monocular Pupillary Measurement

Position yourself directly in front of the patient no further than 16 inches away. Place the spectacle frame on the patient's face and inspect the frame's adjustment. Correct any adjustment problems before continuing with the measurement. Next, close your left eye and ask the patient to look directly at your open eye. Using a grease pencil or a marker, dot the center of the patient's left pupil on the demo lens. Now, close your right eye and open the left. Ask your patient to look directly at your open eye and place a mark on the demo lens in the center of the patient's right pupil. Remove the frame and draw a vertical line at the center of the bridge with your grease pencil. Consider this point to be 0. Measure from the 0 point horizontally to each dot to determine the monocular PD for each eye. These markings will also give you the optical center placement if it is needed for your order (Figure 3-19). (Since you have it, why not include it?)

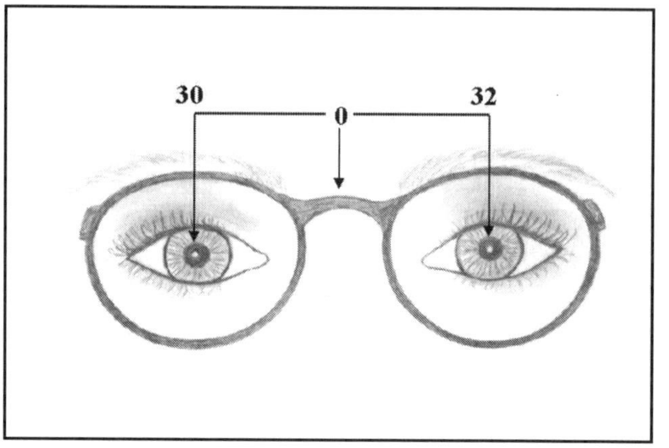

Figure 3-19. Determining the monocular pupillary measurement.

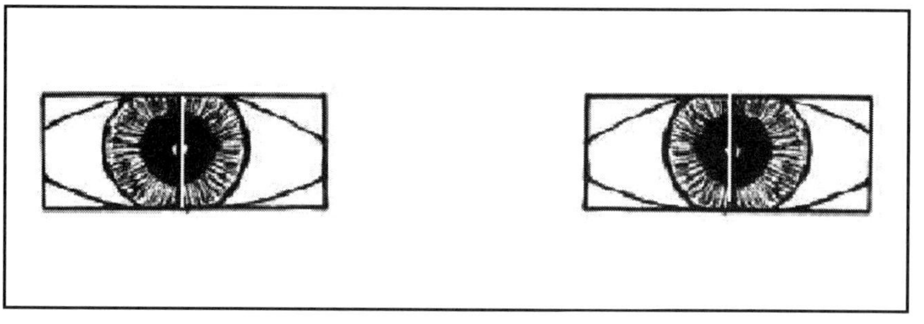

Figure 3-20. The vertical lines inside the pupillometer are aligned with the light reflexes on each cornea.

Measuring the Pupillary Distance with a Corneal Reflection Pupillometer

A corneal reflection pupillometer (CRP) is a mechanical device that most precisely determines the monocular or binocular PD. The accuracy of this device depends upon its calibration as well as the dispenser's ability to correctly locate the patient's corneal reflex (Figure 3-20). (The corneal reflex is the reflection of the light inside the instrument on the cornea.) CRPs should be routinely returned to the manufacturer for calibration.

To use a CRP:

1. Using an alcohol wipe, clean all areas of the pupillometer that come into contact with the patient's face.
2. Ask the patient to assist you in holding the pupillometer up to his or her face. (It is sometimes helpful to instruct the patient to hold the pupillometer as if using a pair of binoculars.)
3. Adjust the knob on the top of the pupillometer to the infinity position (∞).
4. Looking through the eyepiece, move the sliding pieces beneath your thumbs so that the vertical lines inside the pupillometer are aligned with the light reflexes on both corneas.
5. Turn the instrument over and take note of the measurements. The pupillometer will give you the binocular dimension (usually in the center) plus the monocular calculations for each eye (Figure 3-21).

Note: These instructions are basic guidelines. Always follow the directions that accompany your instrument for more detailed information.

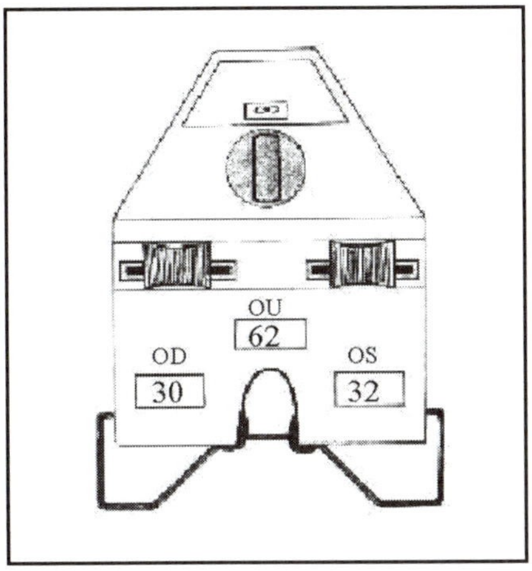

Figure 3-21. Corneal reflection pupillometer.

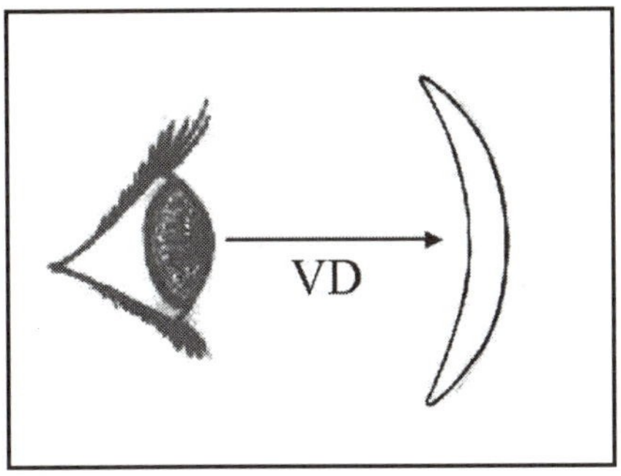

Figure 3-22. The vertex measurement is the distance in millimeters between the cornea and the back of the lens.

Vertex Distance

OptA

OphT

The vertex distance (VD) is the distance (in millimeters) between the back surface of an ophthalmic lens and the patient's cornea (Figure 3-22). A distometer is a hand-held calibration tool that is used to determine this measurement.

When fitting a patient with lenses of +/- 5.00 D or greater, it is important to note the VD that was used during the patient's examination. (It is the prescriber's responsibility to provide this measurement.) The perceived dioptric power of a lens varies if the lens is moved closer to or farther away from the patient's eye. The effective power of a plus lens becomes stronger when the VD is greater than was used during the initial examination. The effective power of a minus lens with an increased VD becomes weaker. Ideally, the VD of the patient's new glasses should be the same as the VD used during refractometry. If it is impossible or impractical to duplicate the examiner's testing VD, the lens power itself may be recalculated to account for the difference. To do this, use the rotary chart that comes with the distometer to figure the new lens power.

Using the Distometer

1. Have the patient put on the new glasses in the position that they will most often be worn. (It is important for the patient to put the glasses on him- or herself to ensure that the placement is accurate. The measurement could be different if the dispenser places the glasses on the patient.)

2. Ask the patient to close his or her eyes. Gently place the stationary foot of the distometer against the closed lid. Do not press on the globe. Slowly press the plunger until the arm of the

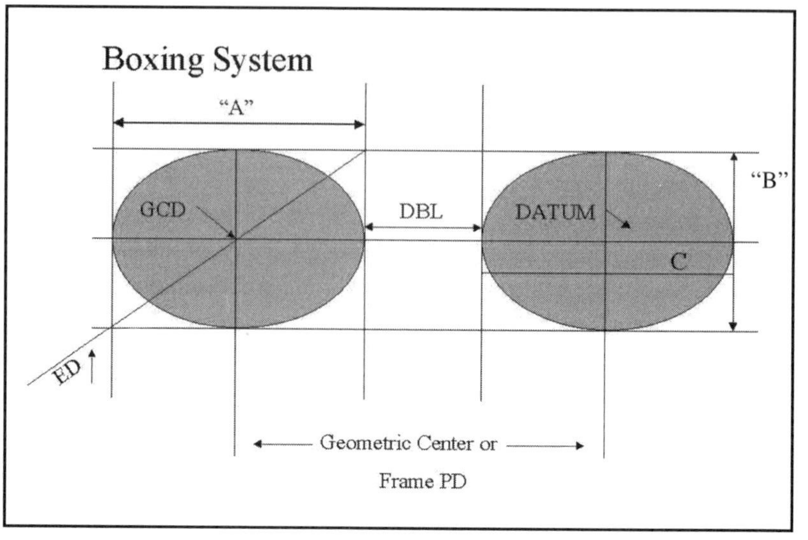

Figure 3-23. The boxing system.

device touches the backside of the lens. Note the vertex measurement in millimeters on the scale. (Make sure that you are measuring through only one thickness of the lid, not folded over tissue. Also, some distometers automatically compensate for the thickness of the eyelid. If your distometer does not compensate for the lid thickness, add 1 mm to the measurement.)

For safety's sake, it is very important to feel comfortable with this tool before using it on a patient. Opticians and technicians may choose to practice on one another to perfect their technique. Most importantly, be sure that the patient's eye remains closed while taking the measurement.

Using the Distometer Rotary Chart

1. Determine the VD that was used during the patient's initial examination.
2. Using the red scale for minus lenses or the black scale for plus lenses, turn the chart until the prescribed spherical power of the lens aligns with the initial VD of the trial lens. (The trial lens could be in either the phoropter or in a trial frame.)
3. Now, without moving the dial, find the VD of the new spectacles. The recalculated lens power is adjacent to the spectacle VD.

Frame and Lens Measurements

OptA
OphA

The Boxing System

The boxing system (Figure 3-23) is the preferred means in the optical industry of obtaining necessary frame and lens measurements. Opticians and laboratory technicians depend on this system to manufacture lens accurately. It is essential to take accurate measurements of the spectacle frame each time an order is placed for ophthalmic lenses.

The "A" measurement refers to the eye size of the frame. Often the eye size of the frame is not exactly as the manufacturer intended. The frame may be stamped 52 mm but may actually measure 53.5 mm. Being unaware of the difference in this measurement could result in lenses that are decentered or ground inaccurately.

Determine the "A" measurement by using a millimeter ruler to measure horizontally inside one of the eyewires from side to side. Add 1 mm to this measurement to account for the groove inside the eyewire. (The groove inside a frame is necessary to hold the lenses in place. Lenses are beveled to fit snugly inside the groove of an eyewire.)

The "B" measurement is the vertical measurement. This measurement is important when specifying the optical center placement or when measuring for a multifocal. Calculate the "B" measurement by using a millimeter ruler to measure vertically inside the deepest portion of the eyewire from top to bottom. Add 1 mm to this number to account for the groove inside the frame.

Many opticians indicate the segment height by using the "B" measurement. For example, an order might state that the bifocal placement is 3 mm below center. To find this location, first divide the "B" measurement by 2. The resulting number is the geometric center of the lens. The bifocal on this order is placed 3 mm below the geometric center of the lens. Example: The "B" measurement of a frame is 50 mm; divide this number by 2, which results in a geometric center of 25 mm. If the bifocal placement is 3 mm below the geometric center (25 mm), then the segment height of the bifocal is 22 mm (25 mm – 3 mm = 22 mm).

The "ED" is the effective diameter of a lens. This is a diagonal measurement from one corner of the lens to the other. This measurement is important when determining blank size. Take the "ED" measurement by using a millimeter ruler to measure from one corner of the lens opening to the opposite edge. Add 1 mm to this figure to account for the groove inside the frame.

The DBL is the width of the bridge. Calculate this figure by measuring the distance between the eyewires at the narrowest point of the bridge with a millimeter ruler. The DBL measurement is also needed to determine the blank size of a lens.

The "C" measurement refers to the datum line measurement, which equals both "A" measurements plus the DBL.

The GCD (geometric center distance) or the "Frame PD" is the DBL added to the "A" measurement. This dimension is necessary to calculate the needed blank size before surfacing or edging lenses for a frame. Take this measurement by using a millimeter ruler to measure from the inside of the bridge, across the lens opening, to the inside of the eyewire close to the temple. Some refer to the GCD as the distance between centers (DBC).

Determining the Blank Size

Determining the blank size before finalizing the lens order is important because some lenses are only available in relatively small diameters. For instance, an occupational segment lens order might call for a 76-mm size blank but the lens is only available in a 68-mm blank. In this case it would be necessary to reselect a frame with a smaller amount of decentration so that the 68-mm lens blank would meet the blank size requirements for the job.

The minimum blank size is determined by adding the "ED" measurement with the total amount of decentration plus 2 mm for edging purposes. The total amount of decentration is figured by adding the "A" measurement to the DBL measurement and then subtracting the patient's PD.

Example: "ED" = 60 mm and the total decentration is 10 mm, plus 2 mm for edging results in a blank size of 72 mm.

Segment Height and Placement

OptA

The segment height determines the placement of a multifocal segment. The type of multifocal segment could be either a bifocal, trifocal, occupational, or progressive (see Chapter 2). If the prescription states that the patient requires an "Add" power, this indicates that the patient needs some sort of bifocal or multifocal to assist with reading or with intermediate needs. (The "Add" power is a plus-powered bifocal segment that aids patients in viewing items within 16 inches for reading, or a trifocal that magnifies objects within 30 inches for intermediate use. If needed, doctors can alter these dimensions to prescribe lenses that will perform at various viewing distances.)

The segment height is given in millimeters and is measured from the deepest portion of the eyewire. The actual placement of a multifocal segment will vary depending on the placement of the patient's previous multifocal and the type of multifocal being prescribed. To best meet the needs of the patient, it is important to discuss his or her lifestyle to select the most appropriate multifocal. Information about the patient's occupation and hobbies will provide insight into the best lens design.

Bifocals

Determine the appropriate placement of the segment by inspecting the position of the bifocal on the patient's previous glasses. Ask the patient if he or she has been satisfied with the location of the old bifocal. If so, match the height of the new bifocal to the old lenses. This measurement is made simple by using a grease pencil to draw a horizontal line indicating the approximate segment position on the demo lenses in the new frame. To do this, place the new frame on the patient, making sure that the adjustment is accurate. Draw a line across the lens with the grease pencil simulating the top of the bifocal. Note the placement of the line against the patient's face. Have the patient take off the new frame and put on their old glasses. Inspect the placement of the old bifocal. Continue to alter the line that you have drawn on the demo lenses until you are confident that the location of the new segment is satisfactory. Then measure vertically from the line to the deepest portion of the eyewire with a millimeter ruler. (Generally, the segment placement of a bifocal begins just beneath the lower lid, or somewhere within a few millimeters of this vicinity.) Never guess at the placement of a multifocal. To diminish the chance of a remake due to segment placement problems, it is imperative to actually draw lines on the demo lenses to determine the best multifocal position. (Please see Chapter 2 for more information about bifocal styles.)

Trifocals

Measuring the segment placement for a trifocal is similar to determining the placement for a bifocal. As with the bifocal, it is important to look at the position of the old trifocal lenses and to determine if the patient has been satisfied with the placement of the segment. Once again, use a grease pencil to draw a horizontal line across the demo lenses to simulate the position of the new trifocal segment. Measure vertically from the line to the deepest part of the eyewire with a millimeter ruler. Most often, trifocal segments are placed somewhere between the bottom edge of the pupil and the bottom lid. Positioning the trifocal at the bottom edge of the iris is recommended because the intermediate and near vision zones can be accessed easily without a great amount of head movement. (Please see Chapter 2 for more information pertaining to trifocal styles.)

Occupational Segments

Deciding on the position of an occupational segment is somewhat more complicated than a bifocal or trifocal segment because the manufacturer fixes the distance (in millimeters) between the upper and lower segments. (This distance varies depending on the lens design and the manufacturer.) As with the other multifocal styles, it is imperative to draw a horizontal line on the demo lens to simulate the placement of the segment. Because of the set distance between the segments, the lower segment is customarily placed slightly higher than normal to allow for a wider field of vision for distance. If the lower segment is placed too low, the top segment will

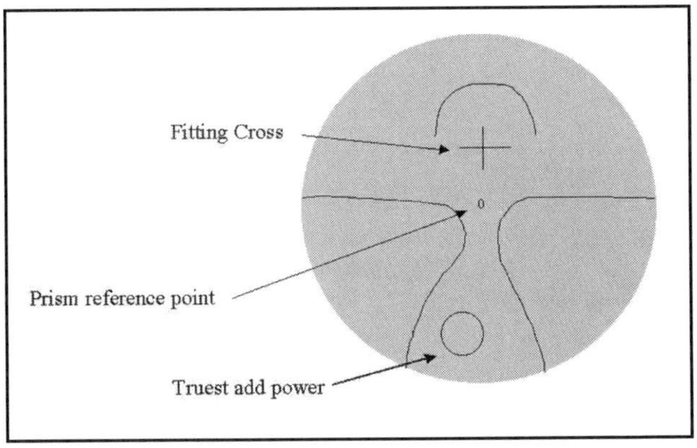

Figure 3-24. Progressive lens.

obstruct the patient's distance vision. (Please refer to Chapter 2 for more information regarding occupational lenses.)

Progressive Lenses

Progressive lenses (Figure 3-24) are aspherically designed multifocal lenses that work like trifocals, offering distance, intermediate, and near vision. When ordering progressive lenses, it is always necessary to include the monocular PD. Using a CRP is the most accurate means of obtaining the monocular measurement. It is also very important for the segment height to be positioned accurately on progressive lenses.

The fitting cross should be centered on the patient's pupils. To do this correctly, use a grease pencil to dot the patient's pupil on the demo lenses. (Follow the guidelines for taking a monocular PD discussed earlier in this chapter.) You now have both the monocular PD and the segment height of the progressive lenses. Use a millimeter ruler to determine the fitting height by measuring from the dot down (vertically) to the deepest portion of the frame. The resulting figure is the segment height to specify on the order.

Progressive lenses should come to your office with the lens markings still intact. Remove these markings only after inspecting the finished lenses on the patient and ensuring that the fitting cross is directly over the patient's pupils. (Please see Chapter 2 for more information pertaining to progressive lenses.)

Optical Center

OptA
OphA

The optical center of a lens is the position along the optical axis where no prismatic effect is found. It is easy to distinguish the optical center with a lensometer by locating the point on the lens where the mires meet.

It is necessary to specify the optical center placement for single vision lenses of substantial power, or when using lens materials with a high refractive index such as polycarbonate or high-index resins. In these particular cases, failure to record the optical center often results in poor vision due to induced prismatic problems. Consequentially, a good rule of thumb is to include the optical center measurement on all single vision lens orders that are over +/-2.50 D. For the same reason, it is also recommended to include the optical center measurement when ordering lens materials that have a refractive index equal to or greater than 1.53. In addition, it is best to include the monocular PD with the optical center height when ordering single vision lenses of a considerable power (or of a high-index material).

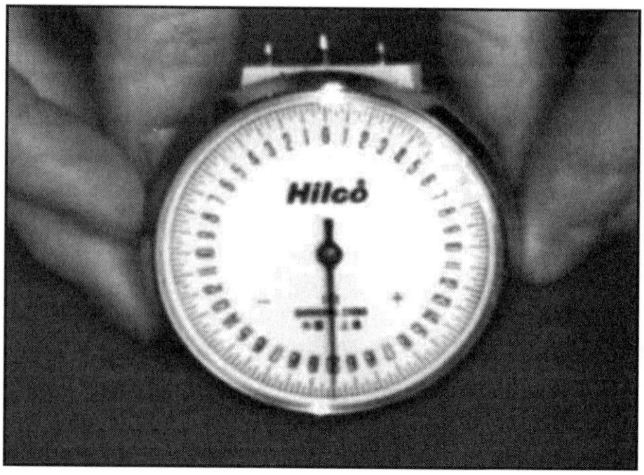

Figure 3-25. Base curve clock.

Taking the Optical Center Measurement

Adjust the frame on the patient prior to taking any measurements. Have the patient place the spectacle frame on his or her face. Using a grease pencil, indicate the patient's monocular PD, then remove the frame. With a millimeter ruler, measure vertically down from your mark to the deepest point on the eyewire for each lens. This is the optical center measurement. The optical center is properly logged on the invoice by writing "OC = (measurement)." For example, an optical center measurement of 24 mm would be entered on the invoice as "OC = 24." This indicates that the optical center for this order measures 24 mm up from the deepest point of the eyewire. Sometimes it is necessary to enter two optical center measurements on the invoice, one for each eye.

OptA
OphA

Lens Clock

The lens clock, also known as the Geneva lens measure, is an instrument used to determine the base curvature of an ophthalmic lens (Figure 3-25). The base curve is the front-side power of a semi-finished lens. After the back surface of the lens has been ground to a particular power, the combination of the front and back surface power results in the overall power of the lens.

The lens clock is a round instrument with three pins located on its base. The pin in the center moves up and down and the pins on either end are stationary. The center pin gauges the base curve of the lens. The face of the clock has diopter powers in red and black. When reading the front curve of a lens, the black numbers are used. The red numbers are used if reading the back curve of a lens.

Base curves are assigned a numeric value by the manufacturer. CR-39 lenses are made on even base curves (8, 6, 4, 2, plano), while high aspherical index lenses are customarily designed on odd base curves (7, 5, 3, 1). To assist professionals in selecting the appropriate base curves, lens suppliers usually provide a reference chart specifically for their lenses (see Figure 2-5).

Patients tend to be sensitive to changes in the base curvature of their lenses. Individuals complaining that objects appear to have rounded edges are describing the "fish bowl effect." This is a common grievance when there is a significant change between the base curve of the old and new lenses. If the patient has a high prescription, keep as close as possible to the base curvature of their old lenses (unless there is a significant change in the prescription which warrants a new base curve or the patient is noticing problems in the peripheral areas of the lenses). Selecting the wrong base curve for a prescription often results in peripheral distortion. For optimum vision, it is always recommended to follow the manufacturer's guidelines for base curve selection.

Using the Lens Clock

Prior to testing lenses with the clock, it is wise to make sure that the instrument is calibrated correctly. This is easily accomplished by "clocking" the curvature of a flat surface. If the lens clock reads zero against a flat surface, the instrument is working accurately.

While holding the lens or glasses firmly in one hand, use the other hand to press the lens clock gently against the surface of the lens (making sure that the center pin is depressed against the lens). To obtain an accurate reading, the placement of the lens clock should be along the 180 degree meridian of the lens (horizontally across the lens) and should not contact a multifocal segment of any kind (flat top or progressive). The measurement is read directly off of the clock face.

Chapter 4

Fitting and Dispensing

KEY POINTS

- Selecting the appropriate frame size and shape can greatly enhance the cosmetic appearance of high-powered lenses.
- The *frame difference* is the difference between the "A" and "B" measurements.
- Patients' visual needs are best met by having a thorough understanding of their lifestyle.
- Anti-reflective coatings provide enhanced vision by decreasing the amount of light that is being reflected from the lens surface.
- A customer response card is an effective means of monitoring the level of service that is provided by a practice.
- Verbal and written instructions regarding the care of the new eyewear need to be given to the patient when the glasses are delivered.
- A good starting place for well-fit eyewear is to align the frame in a standard adjustment.

Assessing Patient Needs

Visualizing the Appearance of the Finished Lens

The edge and center thicknesses of corrective lenses can be altered substantially by selecting a frame that will result in cosmetically attractive lenses. The size and shape of the frame, as well as the fit, significantly influence the final cosmetic appearance of lenses, especially when high-powered lenses are required. Before assisting a patient in selecting frame and lens materials, spend a few moments imagining how the finished lenses will physically look. By doing this you will be able to determine the cosmetic characteristics of the lenses before they have been manufactured. This skill allows you to guide your patients in selecting materials and styles that will result in attractive finished eyewear.

Will the edges be thick or thin? If the edges of the lenses will be thick, will the greatest thickness be at the top of the lens or on the sides? How can the shape of the lenses be manipulated to result in the most cosmetically appealing look for the wearer? Controlling the finished look of the lenses is achieved by making frame and lens selections that will maximize the cosmetic appearance of the lenses while also offering excellent visual acuity for the patient.

Cosmetically Enhancing a Minus Lens

A minus lens is thin in the center and thicker on the edges. The thick edges of a minus lens are accentuated if the patient selects an angular frame or one with an eye size that is too large. When working with minus lenses, a greater amount of decentration will cause a thicker lens edge to be needed (Figure 4-1). The finished lens appears even less attractive if the oversized frame has a square or angular shape. (High minus lenses are *always* thicker in frames with an angular shape, regardless of the lens material.) Therefore, the cosmetic appearance of a minus lens is enhanced by selecting a frame that is a very close fit in eye size and is also round or oval in shape.

The lenses can also be made thinner by using high-index materials. The best way to make a high minus lens appear more cosmetically appealing is to combine a good frame selection with a high-index medium. This combination provides patients with state-of-the-art lens technology and frame styling that enhances the appearance of the finished lens. However, simply ordering a high-index material does not guarantee thin lenses. For best results, combine an oval- or round-shaped frame with a minimal eye size to produce attractive finished lenses. Also, be sure to discuss the extra cost of high-index materials with the patient before ordering.

Selecting a frame style in which the wearer's eye is well centered in the frame (a symmetrical fit) ensures that the edge thickness will be approximately the same at the top, bottom, and sides of the lenses (Figure 4-2). (*Note:* This is not true for lenses with prismatic correction, or for lenses with a large amount of cylinder or decentration.)

It is important to specify the desired center thickness when ordering high-index minus lenses. Verify the center thickness of minus lenses after they have been ground by using lens calipers to measure the center. The center thickness of a minus lens determines the ultimate edge thickness of the lens. The thinner the center, the thinner the edge of the lens (Figure 4-3). Depending on the lens material, the center thickness should be between 1.0 and 2.0 mm (unless the lenses are for safety purposes). The objective is to get the center of the lens as thin as possible so the edge thickness will also be thin. However, dress lenses must still be in compliance with the safety standards specified in the ANSI Z80.1-1995 (see Chapter 2). For the best results, ask your lens manufacturer for center thickness guidelines before grinding lenses.

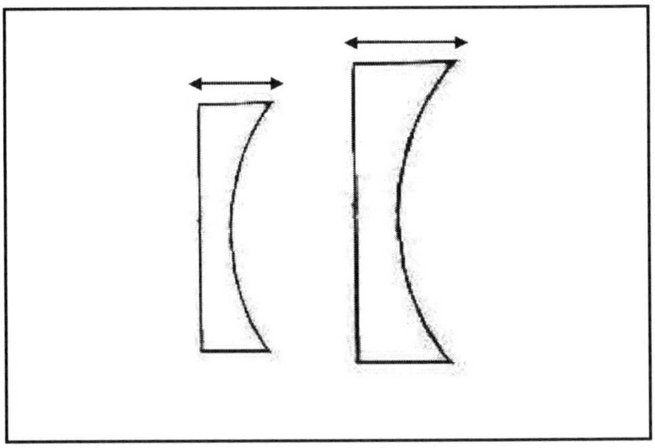

Figure 4-1. The edge thickness of minus lenses is compounded by excessive decentration.

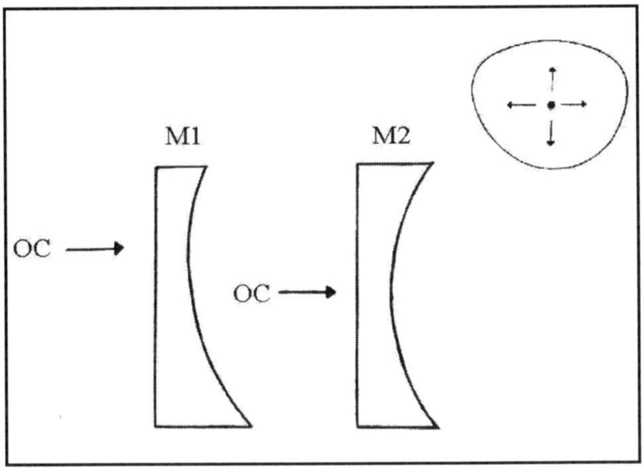

Figure 4-2. Even though the lenses are the same power, the bottom edge thickness for M1 is thicker than then M2 due to the higher OC placement.

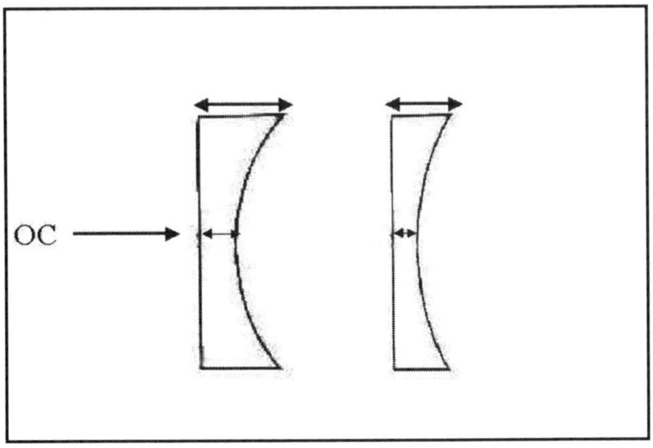

Figure 4-3. The center thickness of a minus lens affects the finished edge thickness.

Figure 4-4. The edge thickness of a plus lens affects the overall thickness.

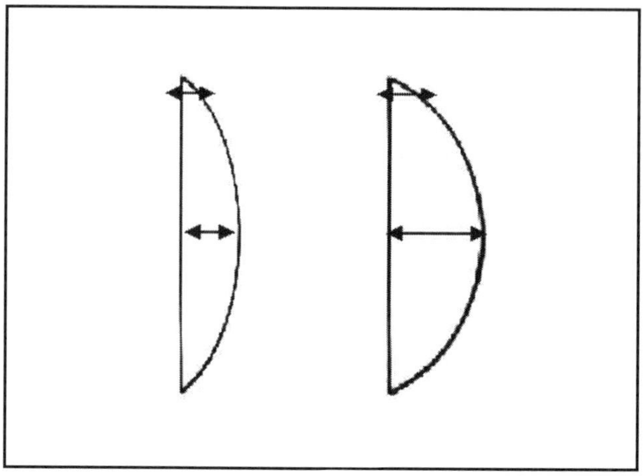

Improving the Look of a Plus-Powered Lens

Plus powered lenses are thick in the center and wafer thin on the edges. Manipulating the cosmetic appearance of plus powered lenses is somewhat similar to minus lenses in that a smaller sized frame produces a more appealing finished product. However, plus powered lenses (especially those of +2.50 D or more) are generally not recommended for rimless style frames because the edge thickness is very thin. When manufacturing high plus lenses for a rimless frame it is necessary to add additional thickness to the center of the lenses. Adding more thickness to the center of a plus lens results in a thicker lens edge. Lenses edged for a rimless mount must be grooved because the frame has a monofilament cord along the bottom of the lens that holds the lens securely in place. High plus lenses *always* look thinner in a full frame vs a rimless design. Selecting a rimless frame for a high plus patient may compromise the patient's satisfaction with his or her new eyewear, even with high-index lenses, because additional thickness must still be added to successfully groove the lenses. A high plus lens mounted into a rimless design results in a finished lens that is thicker than the same prescription mounted into a frame with an eyewire that goes completely around the lens. As with minus lenses, for patients to realize the full benefit of purchasing high-index lenses it is wise to first consider the best frame for the prescription.

It is important to verify the edge thickness of all finished plus powered high-index lenses. The edge thickness of a plus lens affects its center thickness (Figure 4-4). When using the lens calipers to verify the edge thickness of plus lenses, measure the thinnest point of the lens edge. This is usually along the "ED" measurement at the bottom edge of the eyewire. Sometimes it is necessary to check several locations of the lens edge to find the thinnest point. If the lens edge is thicker than 1.8 mm, ask your lab if the lenses can be ground thinner.

Aspheric designs offer the best vision as well as the most cosmetically appealing lenses for high plus patients (see Chapter 2). Aspheric lenses are mathematically enhanced in the periphery to provide better vision for the wearer (Figure 4-5). Not only do the lenses look flatter and thinner, but the wearer also appreciates a broader visual field due to the enhanced peripheral design of the lenses. Aspheric lenses are fit very closely to the patient to maximize the visual field. Frames with nose pads are a good idea because they allow the lenses to fit closely to the eyes. Fitting the lenses closer also magnifies the wearer's eye less, resulting in a more natural look for the patient. It is recommended to offer aspheric lenses to plus- or minus-powered patients with prescriptions of 2.50 D or more.

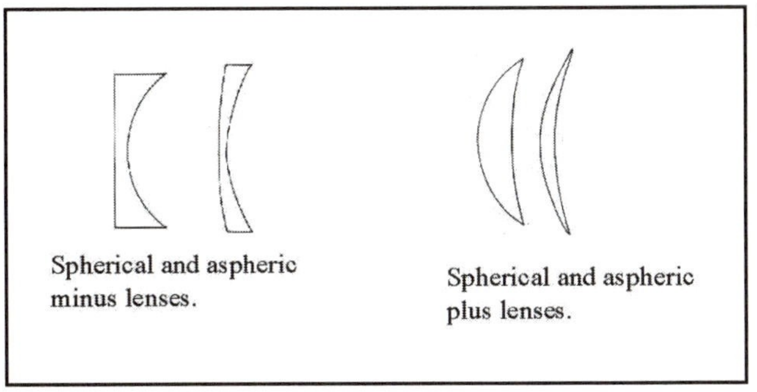

Figure 4-5. Aspheric lenses.

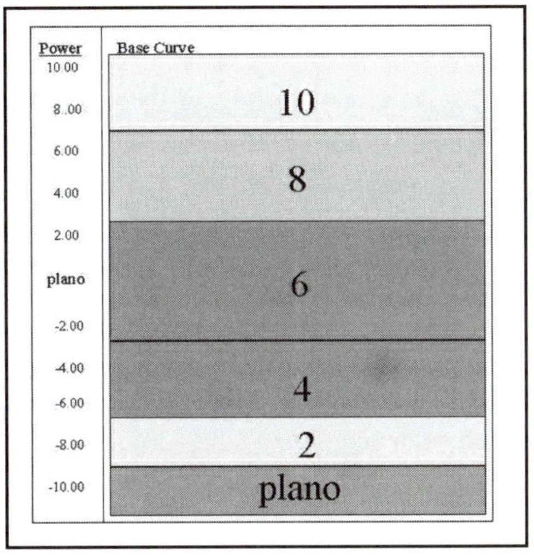

Figure 4-6. Example of a base curve chart.

Patients should be forewarned of possible adaptation difficulties when changing from spherical base curves to aspheric curves. Common complaints after changing to aspheric lenses are:

- Depth perception problems
- A "fish bowl" effect in which objects appear to be rounded
- Enhanced chromatic aberration problems
- A "down-hill" effect in which the patient's field of vision seems to slant downward

Few patients experience these outcomes with their new lenses. Those who encounter these symptoms generally adapt to the new lenses within a few days. For best results, unless there is a significant change in the prescription, stay within 1 D of the original base curve of the patient's old lenses.

It is always recommended to follow the manufacturer's base curve guidelines when ordering or manufacturing lenses. Manufacturers specify base curves for particular power ranges to provide excellent vision as well as appealing lenses (Figure 4-6). Selecting the wrong base curve for a prescription could result in off-axis viewing problems for the patient such as distortion, cylinder aberration, and spherical aberration. Rather than just matching the base curve of the old lenses, research the most appropriate base curve for the prescription by seeking assistance from your wholesale laboratory or by inspecting base curve charts provided by the lens manufacturers.

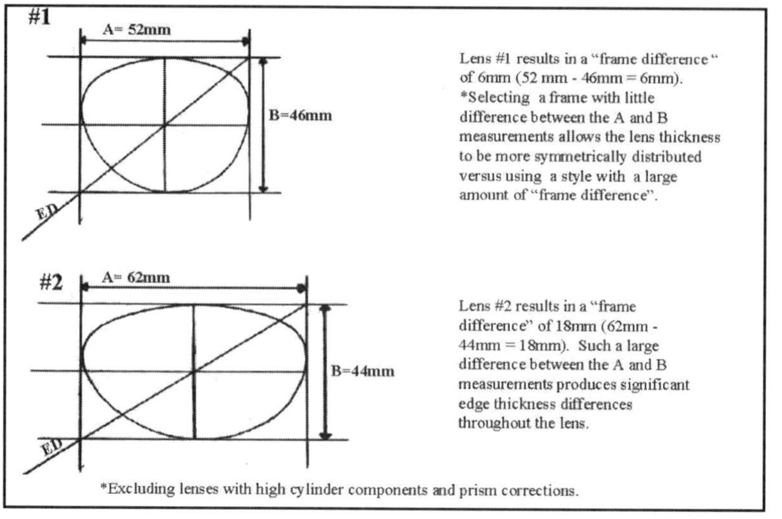

Figure 4-7. Frame difference.

Frame Difference

When manipulating the cosmetic look of an ophthalmic lens, particularly for a patient who requires a high powered prescription, it is extremely important for the frame to have little *frame difference*. The frame difference is the difference between the "A" and the "B" measurements (see Figure 3-13). The "A" measurement is considered to be the true eye size of the frame. The "B" measurement is the vertical measurement of the frame. The amount of frame difference influences the position and degree of the lens thickness. The overall cosmetic look of the finished lenses is greatly enhanced if the frame difference is kept to a minimum. This measurement, along with the position of the wearer's eyes behind the lenses, determines the symmetry of the lens' thickness. If the frame offers little frame difference, the resulting edge thickness will be somewhat equally balanced at the top, bottom, and sides of the lenses (unless the prescription has a prismatic correction or a high cylindrical correction). Positioning the patient's eye in the center of the lens by adjusting the frame and marking the optical center *before* the lenses are manufactured maximizes this technique of balancing the lens edge thickness. Another way to think of this fitting technique is to keep the peripheral edges of the frame as symmetrical as possible in relation to the patient's pupils. (In other words, try to find a frame that allows the top, bottom, and sides of the frame to be approximately the same distance away from the patient's pupils.) For example, a high minus spherical lens edged for a frame with an "A" measurement of 48 mm and a "B" measurement of 60 mm results in a frame difference of 12 mm. This lens will appear much thicker on the top and bottom of the lens because the vertical "B" measurement is 12 mm larger than the "A" measurement. However, if the "A" measurement was 48 mm and the "B" measurement was 51 mm the frame difference would only be 3 mm. In this case, the finished lens would appear more symmetrical in thickness on all lens edges, resulting in a more appealing cosmetic appearance for the (Figure 4-7).

Meeting Your Patient's Visual Demands

Patients' visual demands are determined by their lifestyle. When considering the lifestyle of a patient, we are challenged with selecting frame and lens materials that will meet the visual needs of his or her occupation and hobbies. Selecting appropriate materials and designs becomes especially difficult when considering spectacles for presbyopic patients. There are many different multifocal lens designs on the market and they each meet unique objectives.

When assisting patients with eyewear decisions it is impossible to provide them with professional care without first inquiring about their occupation and hobbies. It is imperative to obtain a thorough understanding of how patients use their eyes and what they expect of the new eyewear. The only way of obtaining this information is by asking questions pertaining to the patient's lifestyle or by including a questionnaire in the new patient paperwork. Either way, this knowledge is meaningful. It is a good idea to write your findings at the top of the optical invoice for future reference or as a reminder while working with the patient. (A thorough understanding of the patient's occupation and hobbies also proves beneficial when considering multiple pair purchases for the wearer.)

A wide flat-top segment would be a good lens design for someone who requires a large reading field due to his or her occupation, such as an architect or draftsperson. However, this bifocal style would not be very appropriate for an advanced presbyope who primarily works on a computer most of the day. This person could best benefit from either a progressive lens that offers a wide intermediate zone or a trifocal style segment. Selecting either of these lens designs would assist the patient with intermediate vision.

Here is another example: A high minus presbyopic patient visits your office to inquire about lenses. After some discussion, she tells you that she is a secretary. Her job primarily consists of working on a computer. While talking with the patient, you learn that she suffers from glare problems when driving at night. Also, she explains that the cosmetic appearance of her lenses is important to her as well as the overall weight of the glasses. By discussing her occupation and by understanding her expectations of the new glasses, we could suggest the following materials and designs to meet her visual and lifestyle demands.

A high-index progressive lens design with a wide intermediate zone would provide a thin, lightweight finished lens as well as good vision for her when she is working on the computer. Adding an anti-reflective coating to the lens would diminish her night driving glare problems while also boosting the amount of visible light being transmitted through the lens. (Anti-reflective coating is beneficial when using high-index lenses because the materials and designs tend to reflect a higher percentage of light due to the density of the resins and the flatness of the base curves. Adding anti-reflective coating to high-index lenses allows more light to transmit through the lenses, which ultimately provides better vision for the wearer. Tints and coatings will be discussed next.)

A good frame selection for this patient would be a frame that is soft in shape (meaning one without corners or angles) that would yield the full cosmetic benefits of the high-index material. (High minus lenses are always thicker when edged for an angular frame. A frame without angles or corners would result in a more overall appealing look for the patient.) It would also be important to select a frame that offers a "B" measurement deep enough to achieve the full depth of the segment for the progressive lens (Figure 4-8).

Tints, Specialized Coatings, and Treatments

OptA
OphA
LV

Tinting

Tinting lenses in the office is easily accomplished by dyes that can be purchased from several different wholesale suppliers. For the best results, frequently replace the dyes to produce accurate tint colors. Using filtered or distilled water further enhances the color and absorption of the tints.

Plastic absorptive lenses can be tinted in a multitude of shades. They can be lightly tinted for cosmetic purposes or to offer some relief with glare problems. Light brown or gray tints seem to

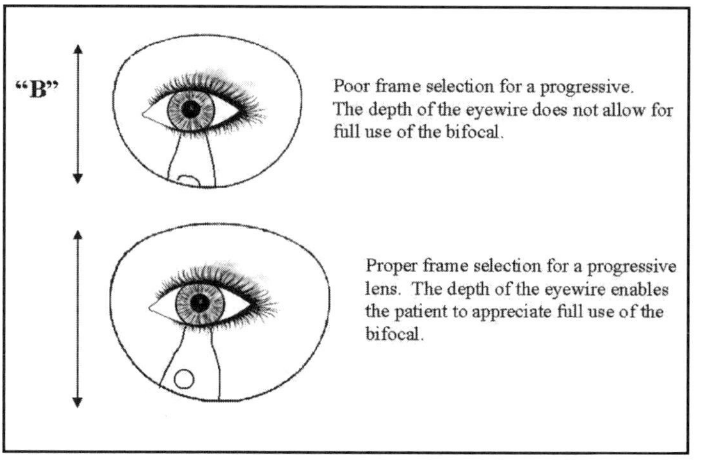

Figure 4-8. Selecting the correct frame for a progressive lens. The "B" measurement of the frame must be deep enough for the progressive near zone.

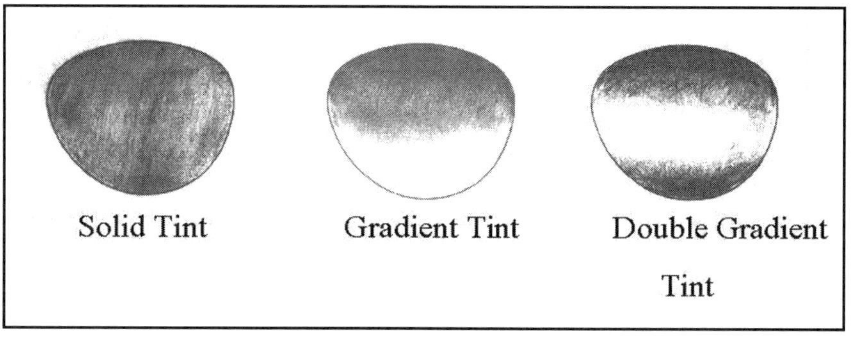

Figure 4-9. Tints.

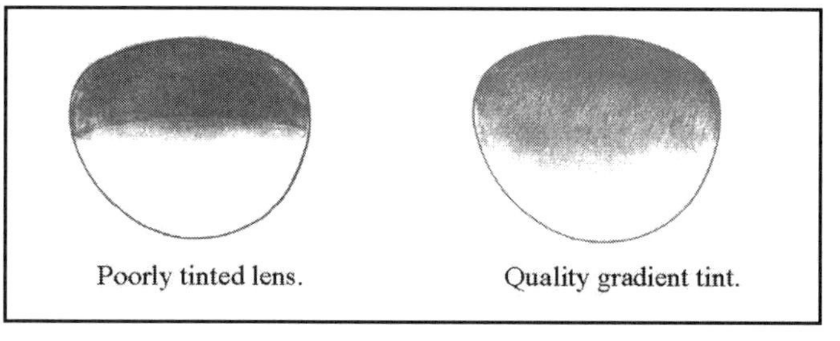

Figure 4-10.

be more effective in controlling glare problems than cosmetic tints such as pink or blue. (However, anti-reflective coated lenses still prove superior in eliminating or greatly reducing glare problems.) Sun-wear depth tints are achieved by allowing the lenses to absorb the dye for longer periods of time.

Lenses can be tinted in a solid pattern, meaning that the entire lens is tinted the same color, or they can be tinted in a gradient pattern that results in the top of the lens being tinted darker than the bottom of the lens (Figure 4-9). This effect is beneficial for bifocal wearers so that the reading area remains clear for near vision tasks. Double-gradient tinted lenses have one color tint at the top of the lens and another color on the bottom half of the lens. Gradient tints are most attractive when the tint gradually lightens to a clear appearance rather than coming to an abrupt stop (Figure 4-10).

Fashion tints have recently become more popular. Patients frequently request yellow, violet, blue, and even green tinted lenses for their everyday eyewear. Likewise, frame manufacturers realize this trend and further its popularity by providing demonstration lenses with fashion tints.

Polycarbonate material generally absorbs a tint of only light to medium darkness. This is because polycarbonate is not a very porous material and does not readily absorb the dye. Overheating or attempting to tint a polycarbonate lens to a sun-wear shade will most likely damage the lens (the surface will split) unless the lens manufacturer has specified that the material will absorb up to sun-wear depths.

The temperature of the dye pots is important when considering the time needed to tint lenses to the desirable shade. Most tints absorb into the lens materials quickly if the dye pots are maintained at a temperature between 175 and 190 degrees. Caution: To avoid overheating, contact your dye manufacturer for recommended temperatures.

The depth of the color of a tinted lens depends on the length of time that the lens is immersed into the dye, the lens material, and the age of the lens. Dark tints are achieved by immersing the lenses into the dye for longer periods of time. A sun tint may require 20 minutes or longer before reaching the desired depth of color. Sometimes lenses tint unevenly; one lens is darker than the other or each lens is a different color, even though they were immersed into the same dye for equal periods of time. This is especially true when tinting a patient's old lenses or lenses that have been in the office stock for some time.

Patients often desire to have their old lenses tinted for sunglasses. Tinting old lenses can result in problems if the they are scratched. The dye is usually dispersed more into the scratches, thus causing the abrasions to be darker than the rest of the lens. Also, always verify that patient's old lenses are not polycarbonate before attempting to tint the lenses. Polycarbonate lenses are frequently destroyed in heated dye pots because technicians are not aware of the lens material. When dropped from a height of about 1 inch above a countertop, polycarbonate lenses make a distinctive high-pitched sound. The sound is similar to that of dropping a poker chip in the same manner. This is a quick and easy test that proves beneficial before tinting old lenses.

Lightening or bleaching lenses that are too dark for a patient may also lighten at uneven depths or colors, particularly high-index or old lenses. To assist us with these problems, dye manufacturers have compiled charts of tips and information to aid laboratory technicians in correcting these mistakes. Obtaining one of these charts and posting it in the lab will provide staff members with the necessary information to correct color matching problems quickly and easily.

Most plastic lenses (including high index) are very porous and tint relatively fast without causing any damage to the lens surface. However, the longer a lens is immersed into a heated dye, the greater the chance of damaging the material. Heat damaged lenses may appear as warped, crazed (the entire surface is cracked), or waved (the surface appears to have melted) (Figure 4-11). These problems present themselves more frequently when tinting high-index or polycarbonate lenses. As a rule, polycarbonate and high-index lenses are more safely tinted if dyes are maintained at a lower temperature and if the lenses are continuously cooled during the tinting process. (Alternately dip the lenses between the heated dye and cool water.)

UV protection, which is important for all sun-wear tinted lenses, is obtained by immersing absorptive lenses into a heated solution of UV filtering chemicals. (Polycarbonate and some high-index lenses inherently provide UV protection due to the material.) Once the lenses are immersed for the required period of time (dependent on the chemical manufacturer), they are capable of absorbing UV light up to 400 nm.

Anti-Reflective Coating

Anti-reflective coating is possibly the most beneficial coating that can be applied to a lens. Adding anti-reflective coating to a lens that reflects a substantial amount of visible light allows

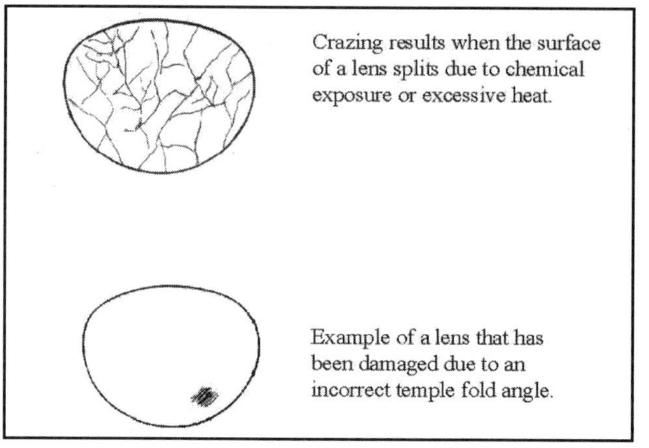

Figure 4-11. Damaged lenses.

more light to transmit through the lens, which enhances the wearer's vision. This thin-film technology consists of one layer (single layer) or several layers (multi-layer) of magnesium fluoride. Anti-reflective coating is applied to the front and back surfaces of the lenses. Lenses tinted for sun-wear are more beneficial if anti-reflective coating is applied only to the back surface.

Anti-reflective coating diminishes the amount of light that is reflected from the lens surface. All lenses reflect light; however, some lenses reflect more light than others. The amount of light reflected from a lens is dependent on the lens material as well as the flatness of the lens (the base curve). High-index lenses tend to reflect more light due to their flat curves and to the high refractive index of the material. With ultra-high refractive index lenses (1.60 and over), it is always a good idea to order an anti-reflective coating so that the patient can achieve optimum vision.

Because anti-reflective coating is superb at transmitting additional light through the lens material, it is best to specify that the lens be clear (ie, with no additional tinting). Tint blocks out light; anti-reflective coating allows for better light transmission. A patient would not realize the full benefit of an anti-reflective coated lens if the lens were also tinted.

Patients should be advised that, unless stated by the manufacturer, anti-reflective coated lenses need to be cleaned with solutions that are approved for this advanced coating. The coating is porous and can absorb materials such as oil or ammonia-based cleansers. After time, lenses that have been cleaned with the wrong solutions appear to have a "rainbow" sheen. (The coating appears multicolored.) However, an anti-reflective coating that appears split or cloudy is defective and should be sent back to the manufacturer to be stripped and re-coated.

Edge Treatments

The edge of heavy or thick lenses, particularly minus lenses, is made more attractive and thinner by rolling and polishing the edge of the lenses (Figure 4-12). Rolled and polished edge treatments are achieved by hand and requested for high minus patients or on drill-mount or rimless lenses. The quality and magnificence of the treatment is dependent upon the skill level of the technician performing the work.

Rolling and polishing the edges of lenses is mostly done by hand. Rolling actually thins the lens edge, and polishing incorporates a buffing machine with polishing rouge to result in an even, shiny surface. A "light roll and polish" means that the edge is not rolled too deeply, this often proves most useable for high minus patients. In skilled hands, the polished edges of lenses with this treatment appear seamless and evenly blended.

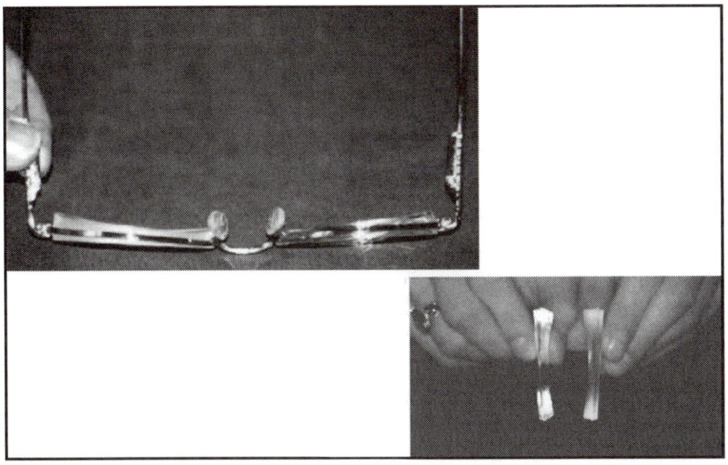

Figure 4-12. Examples of a regular edge versus a rolled and polished edge.

Polycarbonate material is somewhat waxy and does not lend itself well to being rolled and polished (although it can be accomplished). An edge dressing is often used to shine the edge of these lenses. This type of treatment is a liquid chemical that is applied to the edge of the lenses with a cotton swab. Use caution when using this chemical because it is highly flammable.

Discussing Frames, Lens Materials, Coatings, and Options with a Patient

When assisting patients with frames, lenses, and options, it is important to be able to educate them on the products currently available in the optical industry. Lens materials, frame materials, coatings, specialized treatments, and fitting theories frequently change. Educating patients about up-to-date technology allows them to make informed decisions about their eyewear purchases. However, if you are discussing frame or lens materials that you do not completely understand, it is best to be honest with the patient and seek assistance from others for this information. Sometimes you may need to make phone calls to vendors to obtain facts regarding a particular product. Patients are placing their visual needs in your hands; they deserve to receive only the most accurate information pertaining to lens and frame materials.

When discussing optical products, it is always good to have examples of materials on hand for patients to inspect, such as a display that features lens options and materials. For example, high-index lenses could be mounted on one side of a frame, while CR-39 plastic lenses are mounted on the other. This demonstration makes it obvious to the patient that high-index lenses are thinner than CR-39 lenses. A tint display would show the tints that are available, and a frame mounted with anti-reflective coated lenses would reveal the advantages of this thin-film technology.

Handling Patients' Complaints

All optical dispensaries and laboratories make mistakes. For instance, a patient could arrive to pick up glasses that should be ready for delivery only to find that the glasses are not yet completed. Or a patient could visit an office for an adjustment and during the course of the repair one of the staff members breaks a temple on the frame. (To make matters worse, the frame could be a discontinued style!) These situations, plus many more, occur on a daily basis in an optical business. To effectively manage patient care, it is imperative to become accustomed to handling upset patients and transforming an otherwise negative experience into a positive one.

If a patient begins complaining in a normal tone of voice about a situation that has occurred in the office, the most important action one can take is to be quiet and listen. Do not talk and do not interrupt the patient until he or she is completely finished telling the story. Interrupting the patient will only agitate him or her even more; let the patient completely finish the account about what has gone wrong. It is very important to listen carefully during this stage of the discussion so that you will understand the patient's perception of the situation.

When the patient is finished, it is fine to ask more questions regarding the situation to help you fully understand the problem. It is only at this point that you can begin to create in your mind a solution that will change this unsatisfied patient into a happy customer.

If a patient is screaming or talking to you in a very loud tone, it is essential to defuse the situation immediately to avoid upsetting other patients in the office. One method of calming an overly upset individual is to speak to them very quietly, almost whispering. The idea here is that they cannot hear you if they are screaming or talking very loudly. Never take an upset patient alone to an inner office or private area; always have fellow staff members, doctors, or other patients around when assisting distressed individuals.

The goal of any successful optical business is for happy customers to tell family members and friends about their products and services. This way, people who are not yet patients of the business will hear about the exceptional professionals who work in the office and about the quality products that they provide. This marketing technique is absolutely free and is one of the most beneficial means of supplying new patients to the practice. As you may know, it is very costly to advertise in newspapers; word-of-mouth advertising costs the business nothing. However, while happy customers may tell someone about a positive experience they had in your office, unsatisfied patients most certainly will tell others about a negative situation at your practice. Thus word-of-mouth mode of advertising works both ways. This is why it is so important to satisfy even the most irritated patient while he or she is still in the office.

After listening to the patient's perception of the problem, you must try to offer some sort of resolution to the issue. Many times a difficult dilemma can be defused by simply acknowledging the patient's perspective of the predicament while also thanking him or her for bringing it to your attention. After this discussion and exchange of information, it is imperative to act immediately on the matter. You must personally make sure that the problem is resolved.

Utilizing a Customer Response Card

A preprinted postcard that has your office's address on it (as well as return postage) is an effective means of determining the percentage of satisfied customers that leave your office. This card asks the patient to evaluate the office staff, level of service, waiting time, optical staff, and any other items that you wish. The card should be signed by all employees who come into contact with the patient on a particular visit and then given to the patient when the glasses are dispensed.

The dispensing optician and the selling optician could sign their names in the appropriate areas on the card. When the patient arrives to pick up his or her new glasses, the optician could then explain the card to the patient and ask him or her to fill it out and mail it in when convenient. The card enables patients to inform management and team members of satisfactory and unsatisfactory visits to the office. Patients may sign the card or choose to return it anonymously.

When the cards arrive at the office, they should be taken immediately to the manager's office for review. Exceptional cards could be posted for staff members to observe. This is a good way to boost morale among staff members and to bring deserved attention to outstanding employees. Cards expressing negative comments should be given to the departmental managers to pull the patient's chart and discuss the problem areas with the employees in question. Negative and positive response cards could be retained for personnel records and used during performance evaluations, if needed.

If all of the response cards are kept for the entire month, management could tally the overall percentage of total customers by simply dividing the number of unsatisfied visits into the number of satisfied visits to the office. (One might take into account the percentage of patients who do not return their card, as well.) A good target for any optical establishment is to satisfy at least 97% of those visiting the office.

While it may be tempting to withhold a response card from some patients, a practice will only reap the full benefits of this tool if each and every patient is given a card.

Customer Records

OptA

To provide competent service to patients and to comply with state laws regarding medical record keeping, it is imperative to maintain accurate, neat, and easily accessible patient files.

Files should be kept logistically close to the optical establishment to avoid lengthy delays when a file is needed. The charts themselves need to appear neat and orderly. If using manila folders, the patient's name and any relevant information (such as the name of the patient's insurance carrier or labels indicating that the patient is a minor) should be on the outside of the chart. Information on the outside of a chart is always neater if typed instead of hand-written.

Medical and optical reports (invoice copies, superbills, and encounter forms) could be kept in two separate areas or files, or they could be combined in one chart if the optical establishment is part of the medical office. Using one chart for all patient information proves beneficial by having all pertinent reports and invoices in one place. Having one chart with the patient's complete history allows the office staff to spend less time searching for records and diminishes the likelihood of lost paperwork. Lost files result in a loss of productivity for the office staff and greatly affect patient care.

Optical measurements, lens design and materials, and frame information are important aspects of a spectacle order. It is imperative to have a copy of the original optical invoice in order to replace a lost or damaged pair of glasses or to research a problem situation.

Ordering

The optical invoice is a form used to write up the initial spectacle order for a patient. In most cases, this invoice is easiest to use if it is a multiple-copy form and offers a place for general patient information (such as the patient's name, address, and date of order) and the prescription. It should also include detailed information regarding the selected frame style, all frame measurements, the pupillary measurement, the segment style and height, the chosen lens material, and all financial details of the transaction. By using a multiple-copy form, individual copies of the order could be distributed throughout the office to determine financial information for the business, such as sales percentages per employee or for insurance filing purposes. If desired, the optical invoice could also include marketing data to ascertain the means by which new patients became aware of the office. This information is valuable when planning future marketing strategies.

While the office may choose to use a three- or five-part invoice, it is necessary for one copy to remain in the job tray until the glasses have been delivered to the patient. This is the primary copy that will provide information to the lab technicians or to the person placing the order for the glasses.

If the glasses are made in an in-house optical laboratory, the primary copy will need to have all pertinent inset and decentration measurements as well as the base curvature of the lenses. This copy should also include the name of the lab technician or optician who performed the final inspection of the order, indicating that the order was accurately filled. (More on this under Spectacle Verification.)

If the spectacles are to be made in a wholesale laboratory, the office will need an individual who is responsible for placing and receiving those orders. A wholesale optical lab is usually a privately owned, independent supplier that manufactures ophthalmic lenses. In some cases, a wholesale lab may also sell ophthalmic frames and equipment. Most offices, even if they have their own surfacing and finishing laboratory, will need to have a relationship with a wholesale supplier to obtain high powered and/or complicated jobs, such as compound prism or slab-off lenses. For the best turn-around time on lens orders, it is wise to select a laboratory that is logistically close to your office. Most importantly, you should select a lab that offers consistent quality work at fair prices.

OptA

Spectacle Verification

For best results, completed eyewear needs to be inspected by at least two individuals with proven lensometer skills. It is important for both employees to write their initials on the invoice copy to indicate that they have inspected the order for accuracy. The patient should then be immediately notified that the glasses are ready to be dispensed. The invoice copy in the tray also specifies the employee who notified the patient and the date that the call was made. When the glasses are given to the patient, the dispensing optician signs his or her initials and the date on the bottom of the invoice. All of this information is necessary when trouble-shooting problems with the glasses or when researching customer service issues. The primary copy of the invoice remains in the job tray until the glasses are delivered and is then kept in the patient's permanent chart or file.

The following areas are to be inspected for accuracy before delivering completed eyewear to a patient:

- Power
- Segment height
- Tinting
- Lens size
- Safety engravings (when necessary)
- Standard adjustment
- PD
- Segment style
- Coatings
- Lens mounting
- Cosmetic appearance

To ensure that the spectacles are accurate, it is wise to establish two separate final inspection stations. For example, lab employees could be the initial inspectors and the dispensing opticians could perform the second inspection. Both employees would either write their initials on the optical invoice or on a separate check-off sheet indicating that the job has passed inspection. A system such as this keeps inferior product from being delivered to a patient.

Single vision and multifocal lenses.

Meridian of highest absolute power	Tolerance on each meridian (A)	Tolerance on nominal value of the cylinder (B) 0.00 up to 0.75	>0.75 up to 4.00	>4.00 up to 6.00	>6.00
0.00 up to 3.00	±0.12	±0.09	±0.12	±0.18	±0.25
>3.00 up to 6.00	±0.12	±0.12	±0.12	±0.18	±0.25
>6.00 up to 9.00	±0.12	±0.12	±0.18	±0.18	±0.25
>9.00 up to 12.00	±0.18	±0.12	±0.18	±0.25	±0.25
>12.00 up to 20.00	±0.25	±0.18	±0.25	±0.25	±0.25
>20.00	±0.37	±0.25	±0.25	±0.37	±0.37

Progressive and aspheric lenses.

Meridian of highest absolute power	Tolerance on each meridian (A)	Tolerance on nominal value of the cylinder (B) 0.00 up to 0.75	>0.75 up to 4.00	>4.00 up to 6.00	>6.00
0.00 up to 3.00	±0.12	±0.12	±0.18	±0.18	±0.25
>3.00 up to 6.00	±0.12	±0.12	±0.18	±0.18	±0.25
>6.00 up to 9.00	±0.18	±0.18	±0.25	±0.25	±0.25
>9.00 up to12.00	±0.18	±0.18	±0.25	±0.25	±0.25
>12.00 up to 20.00	±0.25	±0.18	±0.25	±0.25	±0.25
>20.00	±0.37	±0.25	±0.25	±0.37	±0.37

Tolerances on the direction of cylinder axis.

Nominal value of the cylinder power (D)	up to 0.37	>0.37 up to 0.75	>0.75 up to 1.50	>1.50
Tolerance of the axis (degrees)	±7	±5	±3	±2

Tolerance on addition power for multifocal and progressive addition lenses.

Nominal value of addition power (D)	Up to 4.00	>4.00
Nominal value of the tolerance on the addition power (D)	±0.12	±0.18

Figure 4-13. ANSI Z80.1-1995 guidelines for prescription ophthalmic lenses.

Verifying the Power, Pupillary Distance, and Segment Height

The power of the lenses, PD, and segment height needs to be exactly as written on the invoice or fall within the ANSI guidelines for the prescription (Figure 4-13). A copy of the ANSI standards for ophthalmic lenses must be available when verifying completed eyewear. This tool is widely used and especially beneficial when verifying lenses that are not ground precisely to the prescription.

Verifying the Segment Style, Tinting, and Coatings

The segment style, tinting, and coatings should be as written on the invoice. The segment width is measured for accuracy with a millimeter ruler. If an optician requested a flat-top (FT) 25-mm bifocal segment but received a FT 28 mm, the glasses must be reordered from the lab. If tinting is requested on the lenses, the tint needs to be exactly as specified or the lenses must be bleached and re-tinted. Attention needs to be paid to lenses with anti-reflective coating. Because the coating is clear, these jobs can easily pass inspection without having the coating applied. A good idea is to use a stamp on the invoice or a flag or sticker on the job tray to indicate that the lenses require anti-reflective coating.

Figure 4-14.

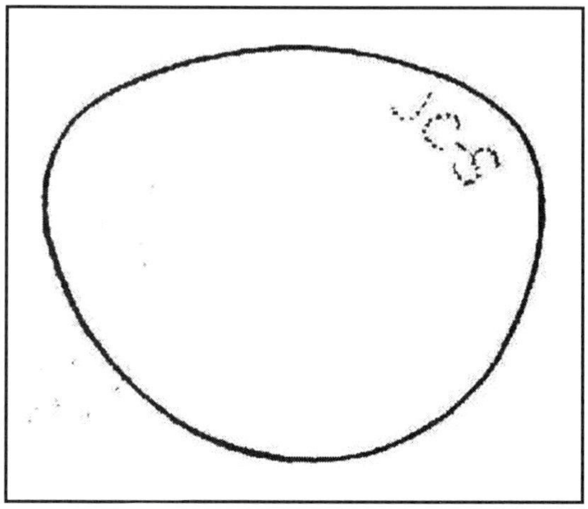

Lenses that are edged and mounted correctly will fit accurately into the groove of each eyewire. Inspect the lens mounting by ensuring that the bevel of each lens is correctly fit into the eyewire. Often times, particularly on aviator frame styles, the bevel of a lens will not be mounted completely in the nasal portion of the eyewire. This could be caused by negligence when the lens was mounted into the frame or because of the power of the lens. (Lenses with a large amount of cylinder correction have steep curves that sometimes pose a challenge when mounting them into aviator frames or frames with a large "ED" measurement.) Lenses that are mounted incorrectly will most likely come out of the frame.

Likewise, lenses are sometimes edged slightly too small which also results in problem lenses, particularly when the glasses are being cleaned. It is wise to check the mounting and size of the lenses before inspecting the power for accuracy. Lenses that are edged too large or too small for a frame must be rejected and reordered from the lab.

Lenses that are edged too large for a frame will cause the frame to have structural problems. If the frame is made of zyl material, the eyewire could split due to stress caused by the oversized lens. Metal eyewires mounted with oversized lenses will have perpetual problems in keeping the screws in the eyewires. Most likely the barrel threads will strip, which means that a screw will not stay in the eyewire unless the barrels are re-threaded. Checking the size and mounting of the lenses saves valuable time for the individual performing the final inspection. It also ensures that the patient receives a quality pair of glasses.

OphA OphMT

Safety Engravings

The ANSI standard for occupational and educational eye and face protection mandates that ANSI-approved safety eyewear consists of a frame that is marked with the "Z87" code signifying industrial eyewear. Lenses, whether plano or prescription, must meet all of the criteria set by the standard. This includes permanent markings on the lenses indicating the lens manufacturer, which is the laboratory edging the lenses (Figure 4-14). This mark is sandblasted or etched into the upper temporal corner of the lenses.

Safety eyewear consists of a Z87 frame and safety lenses; there is no other combination. For example, dress eyewear lenses may not be mounted into a Z87 frame, nor may safety lenses be mounted into a dress eyewear frame. In both cases, the resulting visual systems are not in com-

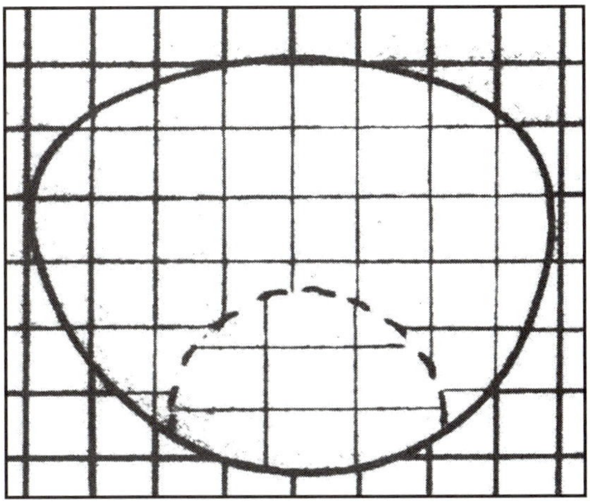

Figure 4-15. Using graph paper to view the near zone of a blended segment.

pliance with the ANSI standard for occupational lenses. A copy of the standard for safety (ANSI Z87.1-1989) and dress eyewear (ANSI Z80.1-1995) is available from the OLA.

Cosmetic Appearance of the Lenses

The cosmetic appearance of the lenses is of the utmost importance to the patient. The cosmetic appearance of a finished job includes inspecting the lenses for scratches, gaps, pits, chips, coating defects, bevel errors, and groove errors. When inspecting the mounting and size of a finished lens, it is wise to also inspect the job for cosmetic flaws. Even if the prescription has been ground accurately, lenses with cosmetic flaws should not be delivered to a patient.

Cosmetic flaws could be caused by equipment or laboratory technician error. If delivered to a patient, these flaws could cause a multitude of visual problems. For example, a pit or chip on the segment line of a FT bifocal could result in reading difficulties for a patient due to unwanted glare or reflections. Damaged or chipped lenses, especially glass lenses, can pose a significant threat to the safety of the wearer. Another example of a lens flaw is an uneven bevel. Bevel problems occur if the lens shifts in the equipment while edging. A lens with an uneven bevel will cause significant problems for the wearer by constantly falling out of the frame, especially if edged for a metal frame.

Some lens flaws, particularly those that are within the material itself, are difficult to detect. An example of such a defect is a "wrinkle" in a lens. This is either a horizontal or vertical error that is within the resin. The best way to detect such a defect is to view a very detailed piece of paper, such as graph paper (or an amsler grid), while looking through the lens. The lines in the paper make the flaws easier to see. Likewise, it is easy to view the zones of a progressive or other multifocals by using this same technique (Figure 4-15).

Patient Instruction

OptA
OphA

Lens manufacturers routinely publish brochures and pamphlets to educate consumers on specific lens designs and materials. This information proves useful during the selling process by first discussing the options with the patient, then reinforcing the information in writing. The OLA offers an exceptional brochure entitled *Lens Menu* that educates consumers about current lens materials, designs, coatings, and treatments. Having these pamphlets available in the waiting

What the Patient Needs to Know

Cleaning instructions for spectacle lenses (without anti-reflective coating):

- Rinse the lenses first with lukewarm water and apply a mild detergent if necessary.
- Gently clean the lenses with your fingertips and rinse well.
- Use an ultra-soft cloth to dry the lenses (a 100% cotton cloth performs superbly without scratching). Never use paper products on any type of plastic lens.

Cleaning instructions for lenses with anti-reflective coatings:

- Only an approved cleaning solution for anti-reflective coated lenses should be used. (If this is not available, rinse the lenses with tap water. Using other detergents or cleansers could result in discolored or damaged lenses.)
- Dry the lenses with an ultra-soft cloth, such as 100% cotton, and use a polishing cloth (usually provided by the coating manufacturer) as a final step in cleaning the lenses.

Wiping the lenses when they are dry causes most scratches. Wiping a dry lens grinds dust particles into the lens surface. To maintain clear, scratch-free lenses, always rinse the lenses well with water before cleaning.

room or offering one to a patient before he or she is dilated increases the patient's knowledge of optical goods. Patients will be more apt to purchase costly lens extras if they are informed about the item and if it is of value to the individual.

Instructions Regarding Lens Designs, Materials, Coatings, and Treatments

During the selling process, patients expect the optician to clearly explain how lens designs function. It is also advantageous at this point to discuss any negative aspects of the design so that the patient is able to make an informed decision regarding lens design selection. For example, when explaining ultra-thin high-index lenses to a patient who has always worn CR-39 lenses, it is beneficial to address the differences in base curvature between the two lens designs at the time of the sale. Ultra-high-index lenses (such as 1.66) have a very flat base curve, usually much flatter than CR-39. Because of this, patients may initially experience peripheral vision problems due to the flatness of the new lenses. Patients are more likely to endure the adjustment period (manufacturers suggest approximately 3 days to adjust to the flatter curvatures) when they are informed about the possible effects that they will experience and when the cause of the problem is explained thoroughly.

Caring for the New Eyewear

Verbal and written instructions about the care of the new eyewear need to be given to the patient when the glasses are delivered. The patient should be notified of the proper procedures for cleaning the glasses so that the lenses and any specialized treatments, such as anti-reflective coatings, are not damaged during the cleaning process. For the best results, advise patients to return to the office for frequent check-ups on their new eyewear. During these check-ups, the screws should be inspected and tightened, nose pads replaced, and the adjustment finely tuned if needed.

Recommending that customers visit your office on a frequent basis also enables you to maintain the eyewear before an untimely situation presents itself, such as a lens coming out of the frame because of a loose eyewire screw.

Instruct children to use both hands when placing glasses on and off their face. The proper technique for cleaning the new eyewear should also be thoroughly discussed with children and their parents. Also, dispensing a hard case with children's eyewear extends the life of the glasses, especially if the glasses are carried to school in a book bag.

Repairs

OptA OphA

Simple repairs that can be handled in the office, such as lost screws or discolored nose pads, are most helpful if they are taken care of immediately. Some offices charge a small fee for replacement nose pads while others view it as an inexpensive means of increasing their level of customer satisfaction and patient loyalty.

Screw-in nose pads, either silicone (soft and pliable type) or acetate (hard plastic), are easily replaced by using a screwdriver with a small blade and snipe- or needle-nosed pliers. Use the screwdriver to loosen the tiny screw (which is holding the nose pad in place) and remove the screw with the needle-nosed pliers. The old nose pad is now easily removed with your fingers. Place a new nose pad in the proper position on the guard arm and reinsert the same screw by using the needle-nosed pliers. Use your screwdriver to tighten the screw into place. Nose pad screws are tiny and come in assorted sizes; they are easily lost when replacing nose pads on a frame. To minimize the chance of losing the screws, work over a job tray or a magnetic pad when replacing nose pads for a patient.

If a patient breaks or loses a temple, either the exact temple or a temporary temple should be placed on the frame so that the customer will be able to wear the glasses. If the frame is out of warranty, or if the patient does not wish to purchase a new temple, a temporary part must be installed on the frame. It is wise to keep a box of spare parts handy for emergency situations such as this.

More complex repairs, such as hinge or solder repairs, could be handled in-house if the office employs a staff member with these skills. Otherwise, the frame will need to be sent elsewhere for the repair. Often local jewelers will repair a solder break for a nominal fee. Also, specialty optical suppliers offer repair services by mail for these and other complicated situations.

Adjustments

OptA

Spectacles cannot perform well without first being in the correct adjustment. Optically, the lenses must be fit at the appropriate VD from the eye for the lenses to provide the same acuity as during the examination. The fitting height of the optical center must be in accordance with the patient's visual axis to provide superior optics, the pantoscopic tilt must be accurate, and the adjustment must be comfortable and secure for the patient (Figure 4-16).

Before beginning to change an adjustment, especially if the glasses were purchased elsewhere, it is important to advise the patient of the risk of breakage. Even in the most skilled hands, there is always a risk of damaging a frame during an adjustment. Please also refer to the section on Frame Materials in Chapter 1 for more instructions for adjusting frames of specific materials.

Standard Adjustment

OphA

A good starting place for well-fit eyewear is to align the frame in a *standard adjustment*. A frame is in a standard adjustment if it has the following characteristics:

Figure 4-16. Correctly fitted eyewear.

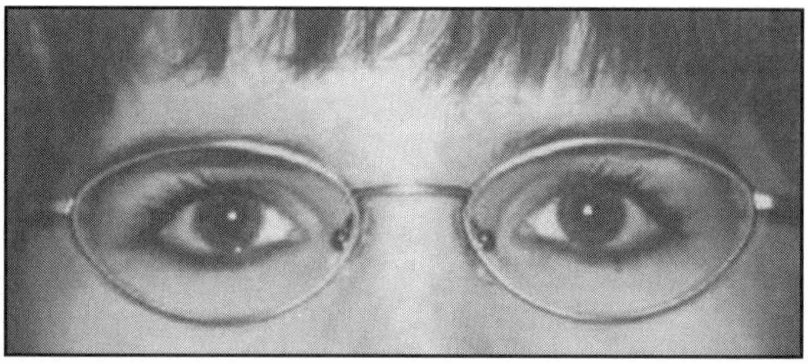

Figure 4-17. Standard adjustment.

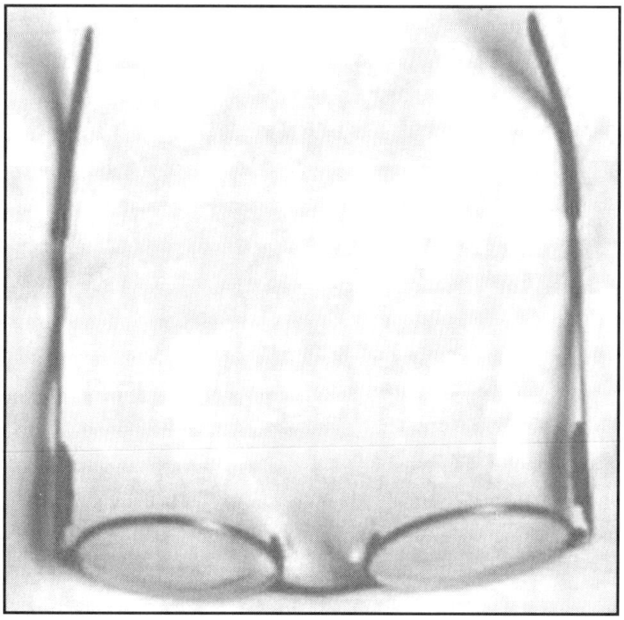

- The bridge of the frame does not exhibit a misalignment called "x-ing"
- A positive face form with vertical and horizontal eyewire alignment
- The temples are parallel to one another, the open temple angle is 90 degrees, and the temple tilt creates a slight pantoscopic angle
- The frame front has the appropriate pantoscopic angle

A standard adjustment or alignment is a "trueing" of the frame. Before adjusting a frame for a patient, it is necessary to place the frame in a standard adjustment. Aligning the frame in a standard adjustment is most often done when the final inspection of the job is taking place (Figure 4-17).

Misalignment of the Bridge or "x-ing"

When positioning a frame in a standard adjustment, begin by working with the bridge. Inspect the bridge of a zyl or metal frame for a misalignment called x-ing. A bridge is said to be x-ing if the frame front looks as if someone held each lens and then twisted them in opposite directions (Figure 4-18). When inspecting a side view of a frame that is x-ing, the eyewires will appear to form an x. The bridge is x-ing if one of the lenses has been moved extremely (or slightly) forward and the other has been moved too far backwards. This adjustment error is corrected by heating the bridge of the frame (if it is zyl) until it is flexible, then moving the eyewires back

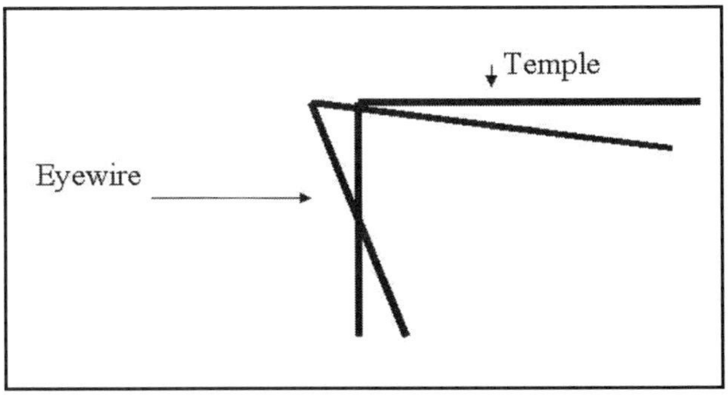

Figure 4-18. Bridge misalignment or x-ing.

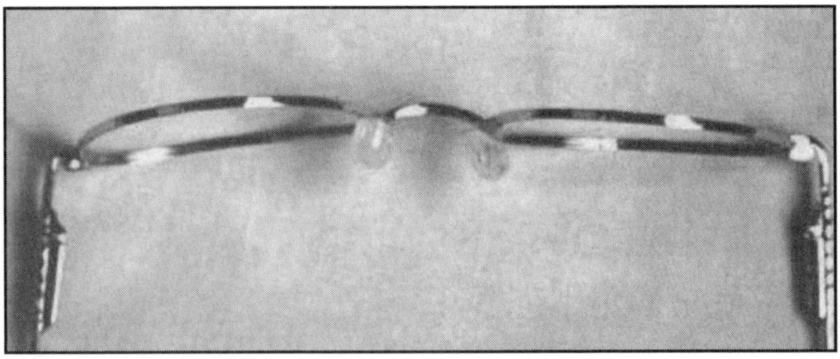

Figure 4-19. Vertical misalignment.

into an even position by hand. If the frame is metal, you will need to use two snipe-nosed pliers or padded pliers for this adjustment. (Padded pliers significantly reduce the chance of marring or damaging the frame while making the necessary adjustments.) While holding the frame at one side of the bridge with one of the pliers, use the other set to move the other side of the bridge into the correct position.

Vertical Alignment of the Eyewires

The next step is to inspect the vertical alignment of the lenses. The vertical plane of the frame front is accurate if both lenses appear even; that is, one lens is not closer or farther away from the face than the other (Figure 4-19). Check for vertical alignment by using the "four point touch test." Place a millimeter ruler on the back of the frame. The frame should touch the ruler at four points: both endpieces and both sides of the bridge. The frame front is out of vertical alignment if the eyewires do not appear to be even. To correct this problem, firmly hold the bridge of the frame. Place your thumbs at the back of the bridge and your fingers at the front (your fingers are placed on the frame where the bridge meets the eyewires). (*Note:* When making this adjustment on a zyl frame, it is necessary to first heat the bridge before moving the eyewires.) Carefully move the eyewires into alignment by maneuvering the bridge of the frame with your hands until the frame front is straight. When making this adjustment on a metal frame, it is necessary to use two pairs of snipe-nosed or padded pliers. One pair is used to hold the frame at one side of the bridge while the other makes the necessary adjustment to the opposing side by moving the eyewires forward or backward until the vertical alignment of the front is accurate.

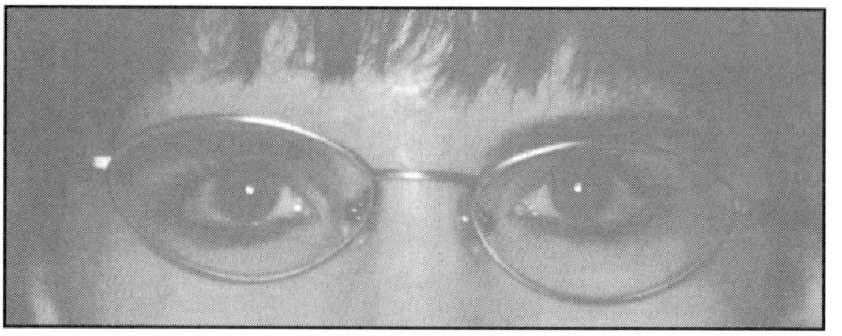

Figure 4-20. Horizontal misalignment.

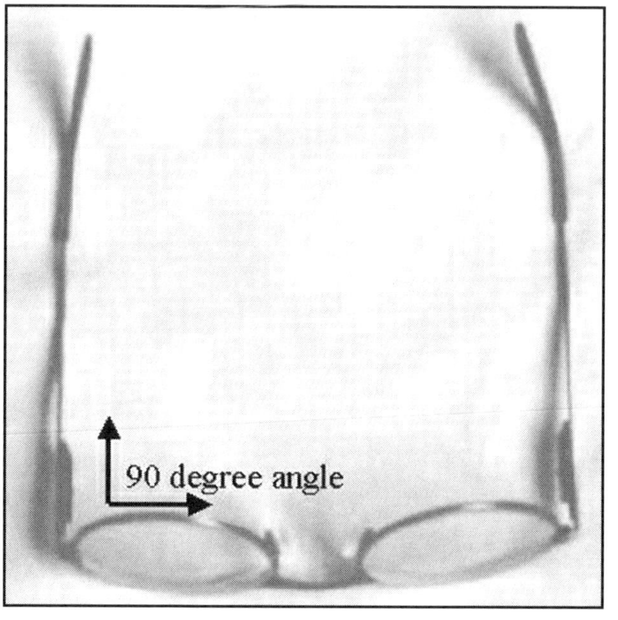

Figure 4-21. Open temple angle.

Horizontal Alignment of the Eyewires

The horizontal alignment is accurate if both lenses appear even; that is, one lens is not higher than the other (Figure 4-20). If one lens is higher than the other, it is necessary to adjust the bridge. If working with a zyl frame, heat the bridge slightly, and when it is pliable, move the eyewires into place by moving them in opposite directions until the lenses are even. If making this adjustment on a metal frame, use snipe-nosed or padded pliers to move the eyewires into the proper position.

Temple Adjustment

A standard adjustment of the frame includes the adjustment of the temples. The temples should be parallel or even when the frame is open. A 90 degree angle should form where the temples connect with the endpieces (Figure 4-21). The temple fold angle should result in temples that do not touch the inside surface of the lenses (to do so would damage the lenses) (Figure 4-22).

Temple Parallelism

Check for temple parallelism by placing the frame upside down on a flat surface. The temples are parallel if both temples touch the surface equally. If one temple appears higher than the other (this can be verified by tapping the temple end; if the frame rocks back and forth the tem-

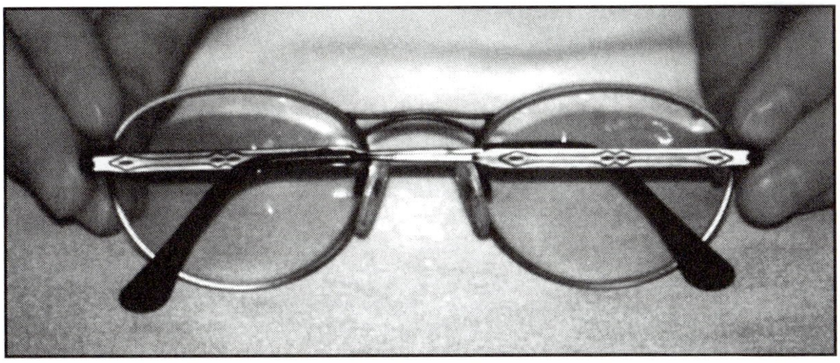

Figure 4-22. Temple fold angle.

ples are not parallel), the frame needs to be adjusted so that the temples are parallel to one another. (*Note:* A large percentage of the general population is not facially symmetrical. Thus, one ear or eye may be higher than the other, or the monocular PDs may be different. For this reason, if a patient has previously worn the frame, and if the temples are not parallel to one another, the "maladjustment" of the temples could be intentional due to the patient's facial anatomy. If the patient has previously worn the glasses, examine the frame on the patient before changing any aspect of the adjustment. This will give you an opportunity to determine if the temples need to be out of alignment to properly fit the wearer.)

Angling the temples is best done without heating the frame front or temple, as doing so could loosen the hinge. Beginning with the temple that is not flat on the counter- or tabletop, use a finger-piece or angling pliers at the hinge to move the temple down in order to bring it into alignment with the opposite temple. An alternative method of determining which temple to adjust is to inspect both temples at the hinges and to move the temple that appears to be most out of adjustment in respect to the pantoscopic tilt of the frame front (discussed later).

Open Temple Spread

When the temples are opened, a 90 degree angle should be created where each temple meets the endpiece on the frame front. Verify that the temples have the correct temple angle by opening both temples and placing the frame upside down on a flat surface. If a 90 degree angle is not formed at the junction of the temples and the endpieces, the temples need to be adjusted. If the temples are set too wide, this is corrected by heating the endpieces of the frame (if it is a zyl frame) and moving the endpieces inward using a padded pliers. If the temples are not wide enough, heat the endpieces of the frame (if adjusting a zyl frame) and move the endpieces outward so that the temple opening will be wider.

Temple Fold Angle

Temples are adjusted with an accurate temple fold angle if the folded temples lie straight and flat across each other and do not touch the inside surface of the lenses. When this adjustment is correct, the folded temples do not cross each other in the middle of the frame; they cross more closely to the center of the bridge. An incorrect temple fold adjustment is corrected by using angling or finger-piece pliers.

Without heating the frame, hold the frame front firmly in one hand and grasp the hinge with the pliers using the other hand. Rotate the hinge until the temple is aligned in the desired position. Check the temples for accuracy by closing them both and inspecting their position. The folded temples should be parallel to one another and should not touch the inside surfaces of the lenses.

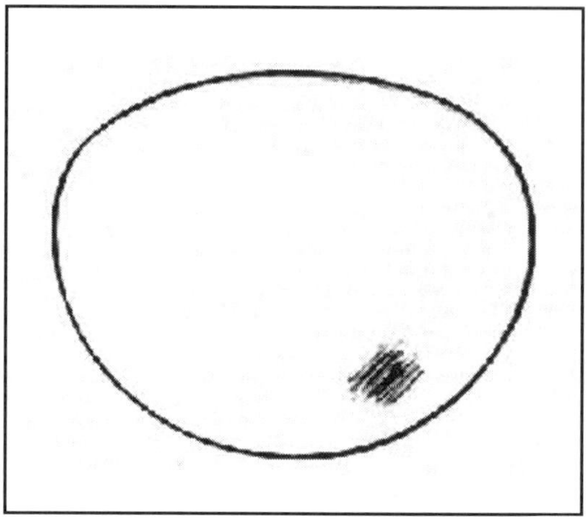

Figure 4-23. Damaged lens due to incorrect temple fold angle.

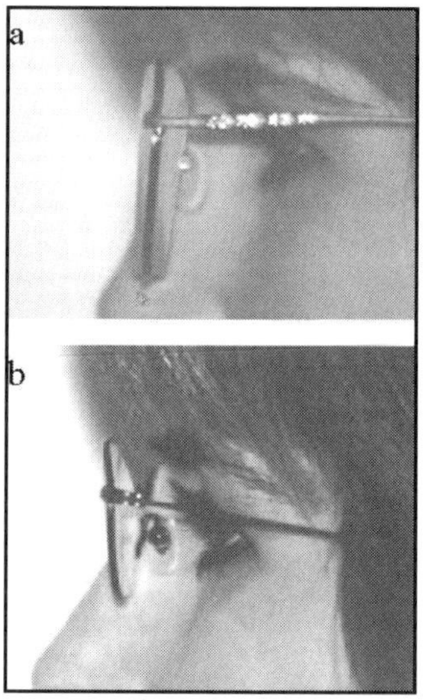

Figure 4-24. Retroscopic (a), and pantoscopic (b) tilt.

After a period of time, an incorrect temple fold angle is easily spotted due to the damage that this adjustment problem causes to the lenses. Lenses that display rubbed or scratched areas in the lower temporal portion of the lenses most likely have an incorrect temple fold angle (Figure 4-23). This damage to the lenses is usually the direct result of an incorrect temple fold angle adjustment.

Temple Tilt, Pantoscopic, and Retroscopic Angle

The tilt of the temples in relation to the frame front creates either a retroscopic or pantoscopic tilt (Figure 4-24). A retroscopic tilt angles the eyewires closer to the wearer's brow. Pantoscopic tilt is the angle created by the intersection of the frame front plane and the facial plane. A pantoscopic tilt angles the bottom of the eyewire closer to the wearer's cheeks. The eyewires should not touch the wearer's face. The desired final adjustment of a frame is for the frame front to have a minimal pantoscopic angle; a common pantoscopic tilt is between 4 and 18 degrees.

The pantoscopic tilt is an important part of the final adjustment because it allows the wearer to experience good vision by properly aligning the visual axis with the optical center of the lenses.

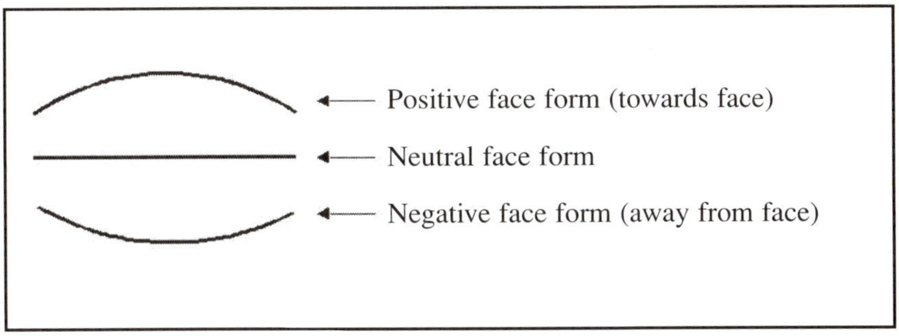

Figure 4-25. Face form.

The pantoscopic or retroscopic tilt can be adjusted by moving the temples either up or down at the hinge with finger-piece or angling pliers. Moving the temples upward increases the degree of retroscopic tilt. Adjusting the temples downward increases the degree of pantoscopic tilt. Either way, the temples should be adjusted so that the eyewires have a slight angle toward the patient's cheeks.

Face Form

Imparting a slightly positive face form to the frame front completes the standard adjustment. A positive face form indicates that the frame front is curved slightly inward toward the patient's face. A negative face form means that the frame front is curved outward from the wearer's face. Frames having neither a positive or negative face form are said to be neutral; the neutral face form has no curve and is perfectly flat (Figure 4-25).

Determine the face form of the front by inspecting the frame upside down on a flat surface. If the frame does not have a slightly positive facial form, an adjustment is needed. (A negative face form or a severely positive face form adversely affects the positioning of the optical centers.)

When making this adjustment on a zyl frame, heat the bridge until it is pliable. With your thumbs on the back of the bridge and your fingers at the bridge front, curve the bridge toward you until the eyewires form a positive curve (toward the face). When correcting a frame that has a positive face form that is too severe, after heating the bridge (if necessary), place your thumbs at the back of the bridge. With your fingers at the bridge front, curve the eyewires outward until the frame front displays a slightly positive facial form. The face form adjustment is done primarily for cosmetic reasons; a frame that bends inward toward the wearer's face is more physically attractive than a frame that is curved outward.

The Fitting Triangle

Properly fit frames touch the patient in only three places: the bridge and the top of each ear. An imaginary line drawn from each point of contact with the wearer's face results in a triangular-shaped form. This important fitting technique is termed the "fitting triangle" (Figure 4-26).

Achieving the fitting triangle for each patient is the goal of every optician. The best means of meeting this challenge is to begin with a frame that is in standard adjustment. Starting with a frame that is already in a standard adjustment, or a frame that only needs minor modifications, guarantees the dispenser that minimal time will be needed to achieve the fitting triangle. If a frame needs to be adjusted extensively, it is likely that the frame did not fit well initially. Frames that fit well require only a nominal amount of movement to attain the proper adjustment. When

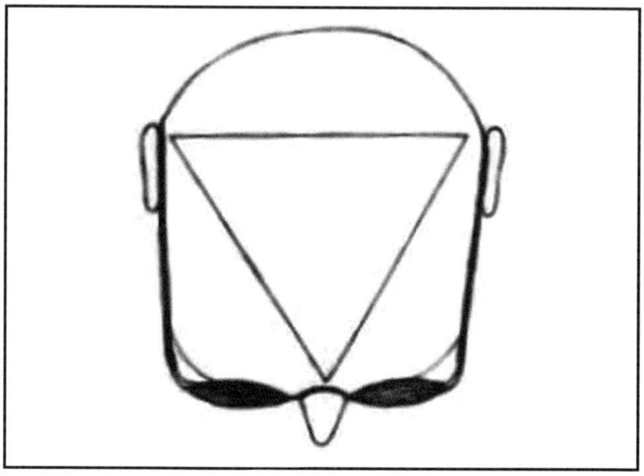

Figure 4-26. The fitting triangle.

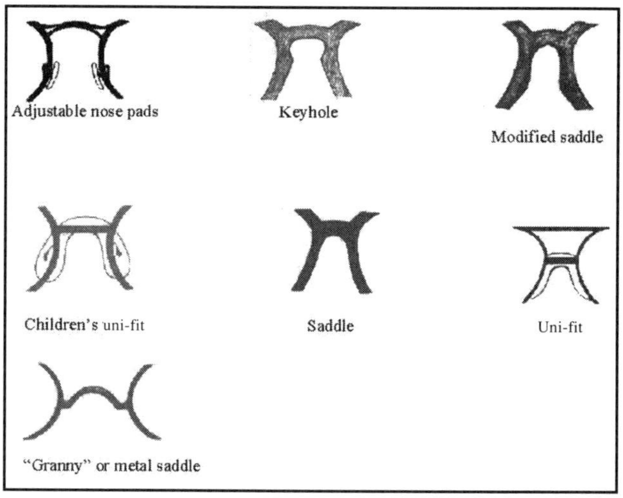

Figure 4-27. Common bridge styles.

faced with a fitting situation that will require extensive adjustments and result in a less than opportune outcome, consider changing the frame style.

Selecting and Fitting the Bridge

The bridge of a frame that is adjusted in accordance with the fitting triangle bears most of the weight of the glasses. For this reason, it is imperative that the appropriate bridge is selected for the patient. The wearer's anatomy, as well as the lens prescription, determines the most suitable bridge design. (This is also discussed in Chapter 1.) A patient with an exceptionally thin nasal bridge will do best with keyhole or nose pad bridge styles. Saddle or modified saddle bridges are more suitable for wearers with an average to wide sized bridge. Because of the ability to significantly alter the adjustment, nose pad frames are suitable for most patients (Figure 4-27).

The prescription is an important factor when selecting a bridge style for a patient. If the prescription calls for extremely high powered lenses or if the patient prefers to wear glass lenses, then the weight of the spectacles will need to be considered. A saddle or modified saddle bridge distributes the weight of the glasses uniformly over the entire surface of the bridge. A keyhole bridge balances the weight of the eyewear evenly on both sides of the nose. Frames with nose

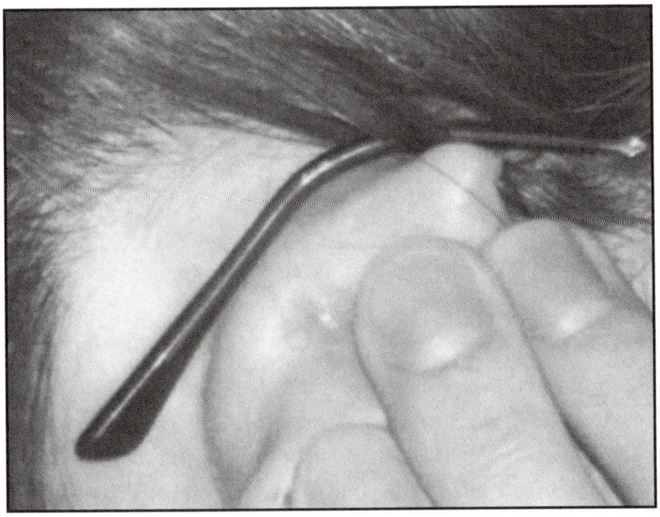

Figure 4-28. The temple end is shaped to closely match the contour of the patient's ear without causing pressure at the crotch of the ear or over the mastoid bone.

pads disburse the weight of the glasses only on the areas of the nose that are touched by the pads. Provide a more comfortable fit for patients who will be wearing heavy lenses by selecting a bridge style that distributes the weight of the glasses over a wide area of the bridge, such as a saddle or keyhole style.

Temple Adjustment

Temples that are adjusted in accordance with the guidelines of the fitting triangle only touch the wearer at the top and behind each ear. The temples do not touch the patient on the sides of the face. To do so would result in a frame that would repeatedly slip forward. Likewise, bowed temples cause pressure at the top of the ears, resulting in discomfort for the wearer. Properly fit temples are very close to the sides of the face but do not touch the wearer until they reach the top of the ears.

The temple end is shaped to closely match the contour of the patient's ear without causing pressure at the crotch of the ear or over the mastoid bone (Figure 4-28). (The mastoid bone or mastoid process is located behind the ear and is an especially sensitive and even painful area for many patients.) Care should be taken to make sure that the temple end is not protruding outward, which would cause pain or discomfort to the wearer's ear. Also, the temple end should not jut too far inward to induce excessive pressure on the mastoid bone.

Adjusting the Vertex Distance of the Lenses

The VD for the lenses should be the same as was used during refractometry (see Vertex Distance in Chapter 3). Altering the VD of the lenses is easily done if the patient is wearing a metal frame with nose pads. A plastic frame or a metal frame with a uni-fit bridge, however, offers little or no means of changing the VD.

An adjustment of the VD is necessary if it is discovered, after measuring the distance between the patient's eyelid and the back of the prescription lenses with a distometer, that the VD of the glasses varies from that used during the examination. (*Note:* The VD becomes an important issue for patients with a refractive error of 5.00 D or more. A common VD used during refractometry is 12 mm.)

If the measured VD is more than was used during the examination, it is necessary to minimize the measurement by moving the frame closer to the eye. If the frame has nose pads, this is easily accomplished by moving the nose pads closer to the frame front using the snipe-nosed or padded pliers. Flatten the nose pad arms very close to the eyewires.

If the measured VD is less than was used during the examination, it is necessary to move the lenses away from the face. Use the snipe-nosed or padded pliers to move the nose pads arms farther away from the eyewires.

Always recheck the VD with the distometer after making any adjustments of the nose pads.

Verifying and Adjusting the Fitting Height of the Optical Centers

The optical center of a lens is the point at which the prescribed power is truest. It is the only location on a lens that has no prismatic power (unless prism has been ground in). In order for the lenses to deliver superior optics, the patient's visual axis must be aligned with the optical center of the lenses. Often times, this means that a monocular pupillary measurement is needed (except for flat-top bifocal segments). Monocular pupillary measurements usually differ from eye to eye.

Use the lensometer to verify and mark the position of the optical centers, then verify the position of the optical centers on the wearer. If the optical centers are not in the correct position, and if the patient is wearing a frame with nose pads, use pliers to alter the adjustment. If the optical centers are too high, adjust the nose pads further apart to drop the optical centers to the correct position, if possible. If the optical centers are too low, use pliers to bring the nose pads closer together, which will raise the centers.

If the patient is wearing a plastic frame, adjust the bridge and either move the eyewires farther apart to drop the optical center of the lenses or bring them closer together to raise the optical center. Plastic frames afford little change in the optical center due to the bridge style.

When all else fails and the optical centers of the lenses cannot be manipulated by adjusting the frame, it is necessary to remake the lenses with the correct optical center placement specified on the order.

To ensure excellent vision for the wearer, it is a good habit to indicate the optical center placement on all lenses and the monocular PD on single vision and progressive lens orders.

Special Dispensing Situations

Occasionally it will be necessary to assist patients who have special needs with eyewear selections or adjustments. Examples of such situations could be a patient who is wheelchair bound or someone who is brought to your office on a stretcher. It could be a patient who has had radical facial surgery or who has been in a traumatic accident. (Dispensers employed by ophthalmologists are more likely to experience these types of situations.) Regardless of the patient's circumstances, it is the duty of the professional dispenser to ascertain the patient's needs and to meet those needs to the best of his or her ability.

In order to restore good vision for these spectacle wearers, the frame must fit comfortably and snugly. A few frame manufacturers will design eyewear for patients with special needs (ask your venders for more information about custom ordering frames). For example, if a patient has recently had nasal surgery it would be important that the eyewear not fit directly onto the nose. The weight of the glasses would cause great discomfort. A frame could be designed for this patient that would meet the new fitting requirements, such as a frame with nose pads that would rest on the cheeks rather than on the nose.

Another option is a custom-made frame called The Multiframe (Priestly and Moore, London, England). The Multiframe offers comfort for the wearer because it does not touch the nasal bridge; it is supported by the brow. It also offers a unique feature in that each lens can be flipped up independently should the patient need to insert contacts or instill medication.

If the patient is hospitalized, wears a hearing aid, or is bedridden, it is necessary to check the temple adjustment to make sure that the temple ends will remain comfortable. Patients with hearing aids require special attention regarding the adjustment of their frames. Often the temples cause the top of the ear, which supports the hearing aid, to become tender and sore due to the temple fitting too snugly between the hearing aid and the side of the wearer's head.

When adjusting eyewear for a patient in a wheelchair, the dispenser should sit directly across from the patient to perform the best adjustment. (A chair with adjustable height is ideal for this.) Standing over the patient while adjusting the frame would not give the dispenser an accurate view of the adjustment, particularly of the frame front and the bridge.

Bibliography

American National Standard Practice for Occupational and Educational Eye and Face Protection, ANSI Z87.1-1989. Des Plaines, Ill: American Society of Safety Engineers, 1989.

American National Standard for Prescription Ophthalmic Lenses, ANSI Z80.1-1995. Merrifield, Va: Optical Laboratories Association; 1995.

American National Standard for Ophthalmics: Prescription Ophthalmic Lenses Recommendations, Z80.1-1995. Merrifield, Va: Optical Laboratories Association; 1995.

Brooks CW. *Understanding Lens Surfacing*. Stoneham, Mass: Butterworth-Heinemann; 1992.

Brooks CW, Borish IM. *System for Ophthalmic Dispensing*. Stoneham, Mass: Butterworth-Heinemann; 1979.

Keeney AH, Hagman RE, Fratello CJ. *Dictionary of Ophthalmic Optics*. Newton, Mass: Butterworth-Heinemann; 1995.

Marco Lensometer Instruction Handbook. Jacksonville, Fla: Marco Ophthalmic, Inc.

Pitts DG. *Ultraviolet Radiation and How to Protect the Eye Against It*. Bowie, Md: National Academy of Opticianry; 1993.

Stein HA, Slatt BJ, Stein RM. *The Ophthalmic Assistant: Fundamentals and Clinical Practice*. St. Louis, Mo: Mosby, Inc; 1988.

Weber JM. *The Eye-Glassery*. 2nd ed. Melville, NY: Marchon Eyewear, Inc; 1996.

Index